MEDICAL PHYSICS HANDBOOK of

Radiation Therapy

MEDICAL PHYSICS HANDBOOK of

Radiation Therapy

by
Ann E. Wright, Ph.D.

Series Editor:
Siamak Shahabi, Ph.D., F.A.B.R.

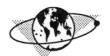

MEDICAL PHYSICS PUBLISHING
Madison, Wisconsin

Published by:

Medical Physics Publishing
732 N. Midvale Boulevard
Madison, WI 53705

ISBN: 0-944838-17-0

Cover design by Rebecca Chapman-Winter

Preface

Handbooks of Medical Physics is a series based on the NBS *Medical Physics Data Book* (1982), which was published in cooperation with the American Association of Physicists in Medicine (AAPM). Written specifically to be used as a quick and easy reference guide, each of the books in this series contains tables, charts, practical equations and formulas for everyday clinical use.

We thank Ann Wright for her efforts in doing what is often a very tedious and thankless job. There may, of course, be errors, and we request that our readers bring them to the attention of the publisher so that they can be corrected in later printings.

I would like to thank Professor John R. Cameron of the University of Wisconsin-Madison and Founder of Medical Physics Publishing Corporation for reviewing the entire handbook series. I would also like to thank Julie Bogle, President and Managing Editor of Medical Physics Publishing, for her assistance and dedication to this project.

Siamak Shahabi, Ph.D.
Madison, Wisconsin
July 1992

CONTENTS

1.0 General Physics

1.1 The Fundamental Units

Most scientific measurements are expressed in terms of one of four basic physical quantities: mass, length, time, or electric current. Standards for each of these are maintained in selected laboratories throughout the world, and are improved from time to time as methods of measurement become more precise.

Fundamental Quantities and Units

Quantity	Symbol	SI Unit	Abbreviation
mass	m	kilogram	kg
length	l	meter	m
time	t	second	t
current	I	ampere	A

1.2 The Metric System of Measurement[1]

The Comite International des Poids et Mesures (International Committee on Weights and Measurements) adopted an international system of units with the abbreviation SI (Systeme International) which are used by most countries in the world. The system contains two special units for radiology and radiation therapy, the gray, which it recommends be used in place of the old ICRU unit "rad," and becquerel to replace "disintegrations per second." It also recommends the use of coulombs per kilogram to express radiation exposure, and the specific quantity 2.58×10^{-4} coulombs per kilogram be stated in place of the roentgen. Likewise it recommends the specific quantity 3.7×10^{10} Bq be used in place of the curie.

1.2.1 SI Base Units

The SI system is constructed from seven base units for independent quantities plus two supplementary units for plane angle and solid angle.

Quantity	Name	Symbol
SI base units:		
length	meter	m
mass	kilogram	kg
time	second	s
electric current	ampere	A
thermodynamic temperature	kelvin	K
amount of substance	mole	mol
luminous intensity	candela	cd
SI supplementary units:		
plane angle	radian	rad[a]
solid angle	steradian	sr

[a]Accepted SI symbol for plane angle, not to be confused with the commonly used "rad," meaning radiation absorbed dose.

1.2.2 SI Derived Units

Quantity	Name	Symbol	Expression in terms of other units
frequency	hertz	Hz	1/s
force	newton	N	$kg \cdot m/s^2$
pressure, stress	pascal	Pa	N/m^2
energy, work, quantity of heat	joule	J	$N \cdot m$
power, radiant flux	watt	W	J/s
quantity of electricity, electric charge	coulomb	C	$A \cdot s$
electric potential, potential difference, electromotive force	volt	V	W/A
capacitance	farad	F	C/V
electric resistance	ohm	Ω	V/A
conductance	siemens	S	A/V
magnetic flux	weber	Wb	$V \cdot s$
magnetic flux density	tesla	T	Wb/m^2
inductance	henry	H	Wb/A
luminous flux	lumen	lm	$cd \cdot sr$
illuminance	lux	lx	lm/m^2
activity (of ionizing radiation source)	bequerel	Bq	1/s
absorbed dose*	gray	Gy	J/kg

*The gray supersedes the previously used "rad" as the unit of radiation absorbed dose.

1.2.3 SI Multiple and Submultiple Prefixes

There is a set of 16 prefixes to form multiples and submultiples of SI units. It is important to note that the kilogram is the only SI base unit with a prefix. Because double prefixes are not to be used, the prefixes, in the case of mass, are to be used with gram (symbol g) and not with kilogram (symbol kg).

Factor	Prefix	Symbol
10^{18}	exa	E
10^{15}	peta	P
10^{12}	tera	T
10^{9}	giga	G
10^{6}	mega	M
10^{3}	kilo	k
10^{2}	hecto	h
10^{1}	deka	da
10^{-1}	deci	d
10^{-2}	centi	c
10^{-3}	milli	m
10^{-6}	micro	μ
10^{-9}	nano	n
10^{-12}	pico	p
10^{-15}	femto	f
10^{-18}	atto	a

1.2.3 SI Multiple and Submultiple Prefixes

There is a set of 16 prefixes to form multiples and submultiples of SI units. It is important to note that the kilogram is the only SI base unit with a prefix. Because double prefixes are not to be used, the prefixes, in the case of mass, are to be used with gram (symbol g) and not with kilogram (symbol kg).

Factor	Prefix	Symbol
10^{18}	exa	E
10^{15}	peta	P
10^{12}	tera	T
10^{9}	giga	G
10^{6}	mega	M
10^{3}	kilo	k
10^{2}	hecto	h
10^{1}	deka	da
10^{-1}	deci	d
10^{-2}	centi	c
10^{-3}	milli	m
10^{-6}	micro	μ
10^{-9}	nano	n
10^{-12}	pico	p
10^{-15}	femto	f
10^{-18}	atto	a

$1 \, mCi = 37 \, MBq$

1.3 Conversion Tables

1.3.1 Length

	cm	m	km	in	ft	mi
1 centimeter	1	10^{-2}	10^{-5}	0.3937	3.281×10^{-2}	6.214×10^{-6}
1 meter	100	1	10^{-3}	39.3	3.281	6.214×10^{-4}
1 kilometer	10^5	1000	1	3.937×10^4	3281	0.6214
1 inch	2.54	2.54×10^{-2}	2.54×10^{-5}	1	8.333×10^{-2}	1.578×10^{-5}
1 foot	30.48	0.3048	3.048×10^{-4}	12	1	1.894×10^{-4}
1 mile	1.609×10^5	1609	1.609	6.336×10^4	5280	1

1 angstrom = 10^{-10} m   1 light year = 9.4600×10^{12} km   1 yard = 3 ft
1 nautical mile = 1852 m   1 parsec = 3.084×10^{13} km   1 rod = 16.5 ft
  =1.151 miles = 6076 ft   1 fathom = 6 ft   1 mil = 10^{-3} in

1.3.2 Mass

	g	kg	oz	lb	ton
1 gram	1	0.001	3.527×10^{-2}	2.205×10^{-3}	1.102×10^{-6}
1 kilogram	1000	1	35.27	2.205	1.102×10^{-3}
1 ounce	28.35	2.835×10^{-2}	1	6.250×10^{-2}	3.125×10^{-5}
1 pound	453.6	0.4536	16	1	0.0005
1 ton	9.072×10^5	907.2	3.2×10^4	2000	1

1.3.3 Energy

	BTU	erg	ft · lb	hp · h
1 British Thermal Unit	1	1.055×10^{10}	777.9	3.929×10^{-4}
1 erg	9.481×10^{-11}	1	7.376×10^{-8}	3.725×10^{-14}
1 foot-pound	1.285×10^{-3}	1.356×10^{7}	1	5.051×10^{-7}
1 horsepower-hour	2545	2.685×10^{13}	1.980×10^{6}	1
1 joule	9.481×10^{-4}	10^{7}	0.7376	3.725×10^{-7}
1 calorie	3.968×10^{-3}	4.186×10^{7}	3.087	1.559×10^{-6}
1 kilowatt-hour	3413	3.6×10^{13}	2.655×10^{6}	1.341
1 electron volt	1.519×10^{-22}	1.602×10^{-12}	1.182×10^{-19}	5.967×10^{-26}
1 Mega electron volt	1.519×10^{-16}	1.602×10^{-6}	1.182×10^{-13}	5.967×10^{-20}

	J	cal	kW · h	eV	MeV
1 British Thermal Unit	1055	252.0	2.930×10^{-4}	6.585×10^{21}	6.585×10^{15}
1 erg	10^{-7}	2.389×10^{-8}	2.778×10^{-14}	6.242×10^{11}	6.242×10^{5}
1 foot-pound	1.356	0.3239	3.766×10^{-7}	8.464×10^{18}	8.464×10^{12}
1 horsepower-hour	2.685×10^{6}	6.414×10^{5}	0.7457	1.676×10^{25}	1.676×10^{19}
1 joule	1	0.2389	2.778×10^{-7}	6.247×10^{18}	6.242×10^{12}
1 calorie	4.186	1	1.163×10^{-6}	2.613×10^{19}	2.613×10^{13}
1 kilowatt hour	3.6×10^{6}	8.601×10^{5}	1	2.247×10^{25}	2.247×10^{19}
1 electron volt	1.602×10^{-19}	3.827×10^{-20}	4.450×10^{-26}	1	10^{-6}
1 Mega electron volt	1.602×10^{-13}	3.827×10^{-14}	4.450×10^{-20}	10^{6}	1

1.3.4 Time

	y	d	h	min	s
1 year	1	365.2	8.766×10^{3}	5.259×10^{5}	3.156×10^{7}
1 day	2.738×10^{-3}	1	24	1440	8.640×10^{4}
1 hour	1.141×10^{-4}	4.167×10^{-2}	1	60	3600
1 minute	1.901×10^{-6}	6.944×10^{-4}	1.667×10^{-2}	1	60
1 second	3.169×10^{-8}	1.157×10^{-5}	2.778×10^{-4}	1.667×10^{-2}	1

1.3.5 Power

	Btu/h	ft · lb/s	hp	cal/s	kW	W
1 British thermal unit/h	1	0.2161	3.929×10^{-4}	7.000×10^{-2}	2.930×10^{-4}	0.2930
1 foot-pound/s	4.628	1	1.818×10^{-3}	0.3239	1.356×10^{-3}	1.356
1 horsepower	2545	550	1	178.2	0.7457	745.7
1 calorie/s	14.29	3.087	5.613×10^{-3}	1	4.186×10^{-3}	4.186
1 kilowatt	3413	737.6	1.341	238.9	1	1000
1 watt	3.413	0.7376	1.341×10^{-3}	0.2389	0.001	1

1.3.6 Force

	dyne	N	lb
1 dyne	1	10^{-5}	2.248×10^{-6}
1 newton	10^{5}	1	0.2248
1 pound	4.448×10^{5}	4.448	1

1.3.7 Pressure

	atm	dyne/cm^2	in of water	cmHg	Pa	lb/in^2	lb/ft^2
1 atmosphere	1	1.013×10^{6}	406.8	76	1.013×10^{5}	14.70	2116
1 dyne/cm^2	9.869×10^{-7}	1	4.015×10^{-4}	7.501×10^{-5}	0.1	1.450×10^{-5}	2.089×10^{-3}
1 inch of water* at 4°C	2.458×10^{-3}	2491	1	0.1868	249.1	3.613×10^{-2}	5.202
1 centimeter of mercury* at 0°C	1.316×10^{-2}	1.333×10^{4}	5.353	1	1333	0.1934	27.85
1 pascal	9.869×10^{-6}	10	4.015×10^{-3}	7.501×10^{-4}	1	1.450×10^{-4}	2.089×10^{-2}
1 pound/in^2	6.805×10^{-2}	6.895×10^{4}	27.68	5.171	6.895×10^{3}	1	144
1 pound/ft^2	4.725×10^{-4}	478.8	0.1922	3.591×10^{-2}	47.88	6.944×10^{-3}	1

*Where the acceleration of gravity has the standard value 9.80665 m/s^2.

1.4 Physical Constants[2,3]

	Numerical Value	Uncertainty (ppm)
Avogadro's number, N	$6.022045 \times 10^{23}/\text{mol}$	5.1
Velocity of light in vacuum, c	2.99792458×10^{8} m/s	0.004
Elementary charge, e	$1.6021892 \times 10^{-19}$ C	2.9
Planck's constant	6.626176×10^{-34} J $\cdot$ s	2.6
Boltzmann constant, k	8.61735×10^{-11} MeV/K	31.0
Molar gas constant, R	8.31441 J /(mol $\cdot$ K)	31.0
Density of dry air (20° C, 101 kPa)	1.205×10^{-3} g/cm^3	
Velocity of sound in air (10° C, 101 kPa)	331.4 m/s	

1.5 Periodic Table of the Elements

The number above the symbol is the atomic weight, the numbers below are the atomic number and the density in g/cm^3 at room temperature (20° C) respectively.

I	II	III	IV	V	VI	VII	VIII		
1.01 H 1 0.0001									4.00 He 2 0.0002
6.94 Li 3 0.5	9.01 Be 4 1.8	10.81 B 5 2.5	12.01 C 6 2.3/3.5	14.01 N 7 0.0013	16.00 O 8 0.0014	19.00 F 9 0.0017			20.18 Ne 10 0.0009
22.99 Na 11 1.0	24.31 Mg 12 1.7	26.98 Al 13 2.7	28.09 Si 14 2.4	30.97 P 15 1.8/2.3	32.06 S 16 2.0/2.1	35.45 Cl 17 0.0032			39.95 Ar 18 0.0018
39.10 K 19 0.9	40.08 Ca 20 1.6	44.96 Sc 21 2.5	47.88 Ti 22 4.5	50.94 V 23 6.0	52.00 Cr 24 7.1	54.94 Mn 25 7.4	55.85 Fe 26 7.9	58.93 Co 27 8.9	58.69 Ni 28 8.9
63.55 Cu 29 8.9	65.38 Zn 30 7.1	69.72 Ga 31 5.9	72.59 Ge 32 5.9	74.92 As 33 5.7	78.96 Se 34 4.5/4.8	79.90 Br 35 3.1			83.80 Kr 36 0.0037
85.47 Rb 37 1.5	87.62 Sr 38 2.6	88.91 Y 39 5.5	91.22 Zr 40 6.5	92.91 Nb 41 8.5	95.94 Mo 42 10.2	(98) Tc 43 11.5	101.1 Ru 44 12.3	102.9 Rh 45 12.5	106.4 Pd 46 12.0
107.9 Ag 47 10.5	112.4 Cd 48 8.6	114.8 In 49 7.3	118.7 Sn 50 5.8/7.3	121.8 Sb 51 6.7	127.6 Te 52 6.2	126.9 I 53 4.9			131.3 Xe 54 0.0059
132.9 Cs 55 1.9	137.3 Ba 56 3.5	1)	178.5 Hf 72 13.3	180.9 Ta 73 16.6	183.9 W 74 19.3	186.2 Re 75 20.5	190.2 Os 76 22.5	192.2 Ir 77 22.4	195.1 Pt 78 21.4
197.0 Au 79 19.3	200.6 Hg 80 13.5	204.4 Tl 81 11.8	207.2 Pb 82 11.3	209.0 Bi 83 9.8	(209) Po 84 9.2	(210) At 85			(222) Rn 86 0.0099
(223) Fr 87	226.0 Ra 88 5.0	2)	(261) Unq 104	(262) Unp 105	(263) Unh 106				

1) see next page
2) see next page

Periodic Table of the Elements (continued)

1) Lanthanides									
		138.9 La 57 6.2	140.1 Ce 58 6.8	140.9 Pr 59 6.5	144.2 Nd 60 6.9	(145) Pm 61	150.4 Sm 62 7.7	152.0 Eu 63 5.2
	157.3 Gd 64 7.9	158.9 Tb 65 8.3	162.5 Dy 66 8.6	164.9 Ho 67 10.1	167.3 Er 68 9.1	168.9 Tm 69 9.3	173.0 Yb 70 7.0	175.0 Lu 71 9.7
2) Actinides									
		227.0 Ac 89	232.0 Th 90 11.6	231.0 Pa 91 15.4	238.0 U 92 18.7	237.0 Np 93	(244) Pu 94	(248) Am 95
	(247) Cm 96	(247) Bk 97	(251) Cf 98	(252) Es 99	(257) Fm 100	(258) Md 101	(258) No 102	(260) Lr 103

1.6 Properties of Selected Elementary Particles[3]

Family name			Particle Name	Rest mass (MeV)	Mean Life (seconds)	Charge (electron)	Typical decay mode
			Photon	0	Stable	0	
L E P T O N S			Electron (e)	0.511	Stable	±1	
			Muon (μ)	105.7	2.197×10^{-6}	±1	$e + \nu + \bar{\nu}$
			Electron's Neutrino (υ_e)	0	Stable	0	
			Muon's Neutrino (υ_μ)	0	Stable	0	
H A D R O N S	M E S O N S		Pion (π)	139.6	2.603×10^{-8}	±1	μ+υ
			(π^0)	135.0	8.28×10^{-17}	0	γ+γ
			K-meson (K)	493.7	1.237×10^{-8}	±1	μ+υ
			(K^0)	497.7	8.930×10^{-11}	0	$\pi^+ + \pi^-$
					5.181×10^{-8}	0	$\pi^0 + \pi^0 + \pi^0$
			Eta-meson (η^0)	548.8	?	0	γ+γ
	B A R Y O N S	N U C L E O N S	Proton (p)	938.3	Stable	±1	
			Neutron (n)	939.6	918	0	$p+e^-+\upsilon$
			Lambda (Λ^0)	1116	2.578×10^{-10}	0	$p+\pi^-$
			Sigma (Σ^+)	1189	8.00×10^{-11}	±1	$p+\pi^0$
			(Σ^0)	1192	$<1.0 \times 10^{-14}$	0	$\Lambda^0+\gamma$
			(Σ^-)	1197	1.482×10^{-10}	±1	$n+\pi^-$
			Xi (Ξ^0)	1315	2.96×10^{-10}	0	$\Lambda^0+\pi^0$
			(Ξ^-)	1321	1.652×10^{-10}	±1	$\Lambda^0 + \pi^-$
			Omega (Ω^-)	1672	1.3×10^{-10}	±1	$\Xi^0+\pi^-$

1.7 Binding Energies of Electronic Shells of Selected Elements (keV)[4]

Atomic number	Element	K	L_I	L_{II}	L_{III}
1	Hydrogen	0.014			
6	Carbon	0.283			
8	Oxygen	0.531			
11	Sodium	1.08	0.055	0.034	0.034
13	Aluminum	1.559	0.087	0.073	0.072
14	Silicon	1.838	0.118	0.099	0.098
19	Potassium	3.607	0.341	0.297	0.294
20	Calcium	4.038	0.399	0.352	0.349
26	Iron	7.111	0.849	0.721	0.708
29	Copper	8.980	1.100	0.953	0.933
31	Gallium	10.368	1.30	1.134	1.117
32	Germanium	11.103	1.42	1.248	1.217
39	Yttrium	17.037	2.369	2.154	2.079
42	Molybdenum	20.002	2.884	2.627	2.523
47	Silver	25.517	3.810	3.528	3.352
53	Iodine	33.164	5.190	4.856	4.559
54	Xenon	34.570	5.452	5.104	4.782
56	Barium	37.410	5.995	5.623	5.247
57	Lanthanum	38.931	6.283	5.894	5.489
58	Cerium	40.449	6.561	6.165	5.729
74	Tungsten	69.508	12.090	11.535	10.198
79	Gold	80.713	14.353	13.733	11.919
82	Lead	88.001	15.870	15.207	13.044
92	Uranium	115.591	21.753	20.943	17.163

1.8 Photon Fluence, Energy Fluence, and Mass Energy Absorption Coefficient as a Function of Energy[5]

Photon energy (MeV)	Photon fluence Φ/X (photons/(m²·R))	Energy fluence Ψ/X (J/(m²·R))	Mass energy absorption coefficient $(\mu_{en}/\rho)_{air}$ (cm²/g)
0.010	11.7×10^{12}	18.7×10^{-3}	4.66
0.015	28.1×10^{12}	67.4×10^{-3}	1.29
0.020	52.6×10^{12}	169×10^{-3}	0.516
0.030	123×10^{12}	591×10^{-3}	0.147
0.040	212×10^{12}	1360×10^{-3}	0.0640
0.050	283×10^{12}	2270×10^{-3}	0.0384
0.060	310×10^{12}	2980×10^{-3}	0.0292
0.080	288×10^{12}	3690×10^{-3}	0.0236
0.100	235×10^{12}	3770×10^{-3}	0.0231
0.15	144×10^{12}	3470×10^{-3}	0.0251
0.20	101×10^{12}	3250×10^{-3}	0.0268
0.30	62.8×10^{12}	3020×10^{-3}	0.0288
0.40	45.9×10^{12}	2940×10^{-3}	0.0296
0.50	36.6×10^{12}	2930×10^{-3}	0.0297
0.60	30.6×10^{12}	2940×10^{-3}	0.0296
0.80	23.5×10^{12}	3010×10^{-3}	0.0289
1.00	19.4×10^{12}	3110×10^{-3}	0.0280
1.50	14.2×10^{12}	3410×10^{-3}	0.0255
2.00	11.6×10^{12}	3720×10^{-3}	0.0234
5.00	6.28×10^{12}	5030×10^{-3}	0.0173
10.00	3.77×10^{12}	6040×10^{-3}	0.0144

$$\frac{\Phi}{X} = \frac{5.43\times10^{14}}{(\mu_{en}/\rho)_{air}\times(hv)}\left[\text{photons}/\left(m^2\cdot R\right)\right] \qquad (hv \text{ is in keV})$$

$$\frac{\Psi}{X} = \frac{87.6\times10^{-3}}{(\mu_{en}/\rho)_{air}}\left[J/\left(m^2\times R\right)\right]^*$$

*Based on a new determination[15] of $W_{air}/e = 33.97$ J/c.

1.9 Energy of K-Edge and Fluorescent Yield as a Function of Atomic Number[6]

Energy E_k, of K x-rays, and ω_k, the flurorescent yield is presented as a function of atomic number Z. The fluorescent yield is the number of K x-rays per hole in the K shell; $1 - \omega_k$ is the number of Auger electrons emitted per K shell vacancy.

General equation governing fluorescent yield:

$$\frac{\omega_k}{1-\omega_k} = \left[\left(-6.4 \times 10^{-2}\right) + \left(3.4 \times 10^{-2} \times Z\right) - \left(1.03 \times 10^{-6} \times Z^3\right)\right]^4$$

where Z is the atomic number.

Fluorescent Yields as a Function of Energy and Atomic Number of the Material

Z	E_k(MeV)	ω_k	Z	E_k(MeV)	ω_k
10	0.0009		50	0.025	0.85
15	0.002	All energy is locally absorbed	55	0.031	0.87
20	0.004	0.15			
25	0.006	0.27			
30	0.009	0.43	70	0.052	0.94
35	0.012	0.63			
40	0.016	0.70	80	0.071	0.95
45	0.020	0.80	92		0.97

1.10 Mass Electron Density, Mass Density, Electron Density, and Effective Atomic Number of Selected Materials[7]

Material	N_g/N_A	ρ (g/cm³)	ρ (N_g/N_A)	$Z_R{}^a$	$Z_{PE}{}^a$
Water (H_2O)	0.556	1.00	0.556[b]	7.16	7.54
Polyethylene (C_2H_4)	0.571	0.92	0.526	5.22	5.56
Polystyrene (C_8H_8)	0.538	1.05	0.565	5.57	5.76
Nylon ($C_6H_{11}NO$)	0.549	1.15	0.631	5.91	6.25
Lexan ($C_{16}H_{14}O_3$)	0.528	1.20	0.633	6.11	6.36
Plexiglas ($C_5H_8O_2$)	0.540	1.19	0.643	6.25	6.60
Bakelite ($C_{43}H_{38}O_7$)	0.529	1.34	0.708	6.06	6.31
Teflon (C_2F_4)	0.480	2.20	1.056	8.35	8.50
Brain	0.551[b]	1.03[c]	0.567[b]	7.01[b]	7.60[b]
Muscle	0.551	1.04	0.573	7.12	7.72
Kidney	0.540	1.05	0.567	7.19	7.76
Liver	0.555	1.05	0.583	7.24	7.81

[a]Based on exponents of 2.0 and 3.8 for coherent (R) and photoelectric (PE) interactions, respectively, e.g., Z_{PE} for water = $[(8/10) \times 8^{3.8} + (2/10) \times 1^{3.8}]^{1/3.8}$

[b]Values for biological materials based on weight fractions given in Section 12 of Reference 7.

[c]Values given are from work of Rao and Gregg[8] and should be taken as "representative."

Note: N_A is Avogadro's number, N_g is the mass electron density ($N_g = N_A \times \overline{(Z/A)}$ = electrons per gram) and ρN_g is the electron density in electrons/cm³. The effective Z/A is computed from $\overline{Z/A} = \Sigma\, W_i(Z_i/A_i)$ where W_i is the weight fraction of the i-th constituent and ρ is the mass density.

1.11 Mass Attenuation Coefficients of Selected Materials at Selected Energies[9]

Photon Energy (MeV)	Aluminum Z=13	Silicon Z=14	Phosphorus Z=15	Sulfur Z=16
		$\mu/\rho(cm^2/g)$		
1.00 - 02	2.58 + 01	3.36 + 01	4.02 + 01	5.03 + 01
1.50 - 02	7.66 + 00	9.97 + 00	1.20 + 01	1.52 + 01
2.00 - 02	3.24 + 00	4.19 + 00	5.10 + 00	6.42 + 00
3.00 - 02	1.03 + 00	1.31 + 00	1.55 + 00	1.94 + 00
4.00 - 02	5.14 - 01	6.35 - 01	7.31 - 01	8.91 - 01
5.00 - 02	3.34 - 01	3.96 - 01	4.44 - 01	5.27 - 01
6.00 - 02	2.55 - 01	2.92 - 01	3.18 - 01	3.67 - 01
8.00 - 02	1.89 - 01	2.07 - 01	2.15 - 01	2.38 - 01
1.00 - 01	1.62 - 01	1.73 - 01	1.75 - 01	1.89 - 01
1.50 - 01	1.34 - 01	1.40 - 01	1.38 - 01	1.45 - 01
2.00 - 01	1.20 - 01	1.25 - 01	1.22 - 01	1.27 - 01
3.00 - 01	1.03 - 01	1.07 - 01	1.04 - 01	1.08 - 01
4.00 - 01	9.22 - 02	9.54 - 02	9.28 - 02	9.58 - 02
5.00 - 01	8.41 - 02	8.70 - 02	8.46 - 02	8.72 - 02
6.00 - 01	7.77 - 02	8.05 - 02	7.82 - 02	8.06 - 02
8.00 - 01	6.83 - 02	7.06 - 02	6.86 - 02	7.08 - 02
1.00 + 00	6.14 - 02	6.35 - 02	6.17 - 02	6.36 - 02
1.50 + 00	5.00 - 02	5.18 - 02	5.03 - 02	5.19 - 02
2.00 + 00	4.32 - 02	4.48 - 02	4.36 - 02	4.49 - 02
3.00 + 00	3.54 - 02	3.68 - 02	3.59 - 02	3.71 - 02
4.00 + 00	3.11 - 02	3.24 - 02	3.17 - 02	3.29 - 02
5.00 + 00	2.84 - 02	2.97 - 02	2.92 - 02	3.04 - 02
6.00 + 00	2.66 - 02	2.79 - 02	2.75 - 02	2.87 - 02
8.00 + 00	2.44 - 02	2.57 - 02	2.55 - 02	2.68 - 02
1.00 + 01	2.31 - 02	2.46 - 02	2.45 - 02	2.58 - 02
1.50 + 01	2.19 - 02	2.34 - 02	2.36 - 02	2.51 - 02
2.00 + 01	2.16 - 02	2.33 - 02	2.35 - 02	2.52 - 02
3.00 + 01	2.19 - 02	2.38 - 02	2.42 - 02	2.61 - 02

Photon Energy (MeV)	Argon Z=18	Potassium Z=19	Calcium Z=20	Iron Z=26
1.00 - 02	6.38 + 01	8.01 + 01	9.56 + 01	1.72 + 02
1.50 - 02	1.95 + 01	2.46 + 01	2.96 + 01	5.57 + 01
2.00 - 02	8.27 + 00	1.05 + 01	1.26 + 01	2.51 + 01
3.00 - 02	2.48 + 00	3.14 + 00	3.82 + 00	7.88 + 00
4.00 - 02	1.11 + 00	1.39 + 00	1.67 + 00	3.46 + 00
5.00 - 02	6.30 - 01	7.77 - 01	9.25 - 01	1.84 + 00
6.00 - 02	4.20 - 01	5.12 - 01	5.95 - 01	1.13 + 00
8.00 - 02	2.52 - 01	2.96 - 01	3.34 - 01	5.50 - 01
1.00 - 01	1.89 - 01	2.16 - 01	2.37 - 01	3.42 - 01
1.50 - 01	1.36 - 01	1.50 - 01	1.59 - 01	1.84 - 01
2.00 - 01	1.17 - 01	1.28 - 01	1.33 - 01	1.39 - 01
3.00 - 01	9.79 - 02	1.06 - 01	1.09 - 01	1.07 - 01

1.11 Mass Attenuation Coefficients of Selected Materials at Selected Energies[9] (continued)

Photon Energy	Argon Z=18	Potassium Z=19	Calcium Z=20	Iron Z=26
MeV	$\mu/\rho(\mathrm{cm^2/g})$			
4.00 - 01	8.68 - 02	9.38 - 02	9.66 - 02	9.21 - 02
5.00 - 01	7.90 - 02	8.52 - 02	8.78 - 02	8.29 - 02
6.00 - 01	7.29 - 02	7.78 - 02	8.09 - 02	7.62 - 02
8.00 - 01	6.40 - 02	6.90 - 02	7.09 - 02	6.65 - 02
1.00 + 00	5.75 - 02	6.20 - 02	6.37 - 02	5.96 - 02
1.50 + 00	4.69 - 02	5.06 - 02	5.20 - 02	4.87 - 02
2.00 + 00	4.07 - 02	4.39 - 02	4.52 - 02	4.25 - 02
3.00 + 00	3.38 - 02	3.66 - 02	3.78 - 02	3.62 - 02
4.00 + 00	3.02 - 02	3.28 - 02	3.40 - 02	3.31 - 02
5.00 + 00	2.80 - 02	3.06 - 02	3.17 - 02	3.14 - 02
6.00 + 00	2.67 - 02	2.91 - 02	3.03 - 02	3.05 - 02
8.00 + 00	2.51 - 02	2.76 - 02	2.89 - 02	2.98 - 02
1.00 + 01	2.44 - 02	2.70 - 02	2.83 - 02	2.98 - 02
1.50 + 01	2.41 - 02	2.68 - 02	2.83 - 02	3.07 - 02
2.00 + 01	2.44 - 02	2.73 - 02	2.89 - 02	3.21 - 02
3.00 + 01	2.55 - 02	2.86 - 02	3.05 - 02	3.45 - 02

	Copper Z=29	Molybdenum Z=42	Tin Z=50	Iodine Z=53
		$\mu/\rho(\mathrm{cm^2/g})$		
1.00 - 02	2.23 + 02	8.40 + 01	1.39 + 02	1.58 + 02
1.50 - 02	7.33 + 01	2.68 + 01	4.53 + 01	5.34 + 01
2.00 - 02	3.30 + 01	1.17 + 01	2.02 + 01	2.47 + 01
3.00 - 02	1.06 + 01	2.83 + 01	4.07 + 01	7.98 + 00
4.00 - 02	4.71 + 00	1.30 + 01	1.89 + 01	2.23 + 01
5.00 - 02	2.50 + 00	6.97 + 00	1.04 + 01	1.23 + 01
6.00 - 02	1.52 + 00	4.25 + 00	6.32 + 00	7.55 + 00
8.00 - 02	7.18 - 01	11.92 + 00	2.90 + 00	3.52 + 00
1.00 - 01	4.27 - 01	1.05 + 00	1.60 + 00	1.91 + 00
1.50 - 01	2.08 - 01	3.99 - 01	5.77 - 01	6.74 - 01
2.00 - 01	1.48 - 01	2.28 - 01	3.07 - 01	3.49 - 01
3.00 - 01	1.08 - 01	1.31 - 01	1.55 - 01	1.68 - 01
4.00 - 01	9.19 - 02	1.01 - 01	1.10 - 01	1.16 - 01
5.00 - 01	8.22 - 02	8.59 - 02	9.11 - 02	9.36 - 02
6.00 - 01	7.52 - 02	7.67 - 02	7.91 - 02	8.07 - 02
8.00 - 01	6.55 - 02	6.52 - 02	6.55 - 02	6.61 - 02
1.00 + 00	5.86 - 02	5.77 - 02	5.71 - 02	5.75 - 02
1.50 + 00	4.79 - 02	4.68 - 02	4.59 - 02	4.60 - 02
2.00 + 00	4.19 - 02	4.14 - 02	4.08 - 02	4.09 - 02
3.00 + 00	3.59 - 02	3.66 - 02	3.67 - 02	3.69 - 02

1.11 Mass Attenuation Coefficients of Selected Materials at Selected Energies[9] (continued)

Photon Energy	Copper Z=29	Molybdenum Z=42	Tin Z=50	Iodine Z=53
MeV	$\mu/\rho(cm^2/g)$			
4.00 + 00	3.32 - 02	3.48 - 02	3.54 - 02	3.59 - 02
5.00 + 00	3.18 - 02	3.43 - 02	3.53 - 02	3.59 - 02
6.00 + 00	3.10 - 02	3.43 - 02	3.57 - 02	3.63 - 02
8.00 + 00	3.06 - 02	3.50 - 02	3.69 - 02	3.78 - 02
1.00 + 01	3.08 - 02	3.62 - 02	3.85 - 02	3.95 - 02
1.50 + 01	3.23 - 02	3.93 - 02	4.25 - 02	4.38 - 02
2.00 + 01	3.39 - 02	4.23 - 02	4.61 - 02	4.76 - 02
3.00 + 01	3.68 - 02	4.70 - 02	5.17 - 02	5.36 - 02

	Tungsten Z=74	Lead Z=82	Uranium Z-92	Absorption Edges
	$\mu/\rho(cm^2/g)$			
1.00 - 02	9.12 + 01	1.28 + 02	1.73 + 02	
1.50 - 02	1.39 + 02	1.12 + 02	6.03 + 01	L_{III} EDGE
2.00 - 02	6.51 + 01	8.34 + 01	6.85 + 01	
3.00 - 02	2.18 + 01	2.84 + 01	3.96 + 01	L_{II}, L_I EDGES
4.00 - 02	9.97 + 00	1.31 + 01	1.87 + 01	
5.00 - 02	5.40 + 00	7.22 + 00	1.04 + 01	
6.00 - 02	3.28 + 00	4.43 + 00	6.45 + 00	
8.00 - 02	7.66 + 00	2.07 + 00	3.04 + 00	
1.00 - 01	4.29 + 00	5.23 + 00	1.71 + 00	K EDGE
1.50 - 01	1.50 + 00	1.89 + 00	2.47 + 00	
2.00 - 01	7.38 - 01	9.45 - 01	1.23 + 00	
3.00 - 01	3.02 - 01	3.83 - 01	4.85 - 01	
4.00 - 01	1.80 - 01	2.20 - 01	2.73 - 01	
5.00 - 01	1.29 - 01	1.54 - 01	1.85 - 01	
6.00 - 01	1.03 - 01	1.20 - 01	1.40 - 01	
8.00 - 01	7.73 - 02	8.56 - 02	9.64 - 02	
1.00 + 00	6.39 - 02	6.90 - 02	7.54 - 02	
1.50 + 00	4.88 - 02	5.10 - 02	5.39 - 02	
2.00 + 00	4.34 - 02	4.50 - 02	4.70 - 02	
3.00 + 00	4.01 - 02	4.16 - 02	4.35 - 02	
4.00 + 00	3.98 - 02	4.14 - 02	4.34 - 02	
5.00 + 00	4.06 - 02	4.24 - 02	4.44 - 02	
6.00 + 00	4.16 - 02	4.34 - 02	4.54 - 02	
8.00 + 00	4.39 - 02	4.59 - 02	4.79 - 02	
1.00 + 01	4.63 - 02	4.84 - 02	5.06 - 02	
1.50 + 01	5.24 - 02	5.48 - 02	5.73 - 02	
2.00 + 01	5.77 - 02	6.06 - 02	6.36 - 02	
3.00 + 01	6.59 - 02	6.96 - 02	7.33 - 02	

1.12 Mass Energy Absorption Coefficients and f-Factors of Selected Materials[5,10,15]

Mass energy-absorption coefficient (μ_{en}/ρ) in m²/kg
(multiply by 10 for cm²/g)

Photon energy (eV)	Air	Water (H₂0)	Poly-styrene (C_8H_8)	Lucite ($C_5H_8O_2$)	Poly-ethylene (CH_2)
1.0000 + 04	4.648 - 01	4.839 - 01	1.849 - 01	2.943 - 01	1.717 - 01
1.5000 + 04	1.304 - 01	1.340 - 01	5.014 - 02	8.081 - 02	4.662 - 02
2.0000 + 04	5.266 - 02	5.364 - 02	2.002 - 02	3.231 - 02	1.868 - 02
3.0000 + 04	1.504 - 02	1.519 - 02	6.056 - 03	9.385 - 03	5.754 - 03
4.0000 + 04	6.706 - 03	6.800 - 03	3.190 - 03	4.498 - 03	3.128 - 03
5.0000 + 04	4.038 - 03	4.153 - 03	2.387 - 03	3.019 - 03	2.410 - 03
6.0000 + 04	3.008 - 03	3.151 - 03	2.153 - 03	2.503 - 03	2.218 - 03
8.0000 + 04	2.394 - 03	2.582 - 03	2.152 - 03	2.292 - 03	2.258 - 03
1.0000 + 05	2.319 - 03	2.539 - 03	2.292 - 03	2.363 - 03	2.419 - 03
1.5000 + 05	2.494 - 03	2.762 - 03	2.631 - 03	2.656 - 03	2.788 - 03
2.0000 + 05	2.672 - 03	2.967 - 03	2.856 - 03	2.872 - 03	3.029 - 03
3.0000 + 05	2.872 - 03	3.192 - 03	3.088 - 03	3.099 - 03	3.275 - 03
4.0000 + 05	2.949 - 03	3.279 - 03	3.174 - 03	3.185 - 03	3.367 - 03
5.0000 + 05	2.966 - 03	3.298 - 03	3.195 - 03	3.205 - 03	3.389 - 03
6.0000 + 05	2.952 - 03	3.284 - 03	3.181 - 03	3.191 - 03	3.375 - 03
8.0000 + 05	2.882 - 03	3.205 - 03	3.106 - 03	3.115 - 03	3.295 - 03
1.0000 + 06	2.787 - 03	3.100 - 03	3.005 - 03	3.014 - 03	3.188 - 03
1.5000 + 06	2.545 - 03	2.831 - 03	2.744 - 03	2.752 - 03	2.911 - 03
2.0000 + 06	2.342 - 03	2.604 - 03	2.522 - 03	2.530 - 03	2.675 - 03
3.0000 + 06	2.055 - 03	2.279 - 03	2.196 - 03	2.208 - 03	2.325 - 03
4.0000 + 06	1.868 - 03	2.064 - 03	1.978 - 03	1.993 - 03	2.089 - 03
5.0000 + 06	1.739 - 03	1.914 - 03	1.822 - 03	1.842 - 03	1.919 - 03
6.0000 + 06	1.646 - 03	1.805 - 03	1.707 - 03	1.730 - 03	1.793 - 03
8.0000 + 06	1.522 - 03	1.658 - 03	1.548 - 03	1.578 - 03	1.618 - 03
1.0000 + 07	1.445 - 03	1.565 - 03	1.455 - 03	1.480 - 03	1.503 - 03
1.5000 + 07	1.347 - 03	1.440 - 03	1.302 - 03	1.346 - 03	1.341 - 03
2.0000 + 07	1.306 - 03	1.384 - 03	1.233 - 03	1.284 - 03	1.206 - 03

1.12 Mass Energy Absorption Coefficients and f-Factors of Selected Materials[5,10,15] (continued)

Photon Energy (eV)	Bakelite $(C_{43}H_{38}O_7)$	Compact Bone	Muscle	Water	Compact Bone	Muscle
			f-Factors			
1.0000 + 04	2.467 - 01	1.900 + 00	0.496 + 00	0.912	3.54	0.925
1.5000 + 04	6.741 - 02	0.589 + 00	0.136 + 00	0.889	3.97	0.916
2.0000 + 04	2.692 - 02	0.251 + 00	0.544 - 01	0.881	4.23	0.916
3.0000 + 04	7.904 - 03	0.743 - 01	0.154 - 01	0.869	4.39	0.910
4.0000 + 04	3.898 - 03	0.305 - 01	0.677 - 02	0.878	4.14	0.919
5.0000 + 04	2.711 - 03	0.158 - 01	0.409 - 02	0.892	3.58	0.926
6.0000 + 04	2.316 - 03	0.979 - 02	0.312 - 02	0.905	2.91	0.929
8.0000 + 04	2.191 - 03	0.520 - 02	0.255 - 02	0.932	1.91	0.930
1.0000 + 05	2.288 - 03	0.386 - 02	0.252 - 02	0.948	1.45	0.918
1.5000 + 05	2.593 - 03	0.304 - 02	0.276 - 02	0.962	1.05	0.956
2.0000 + 05	2.808 - 03	0.302 - 02	0.297 - 02	0.973	0.979	0.983
3.0000 + 05	3.032 - 03	0.311 - 02	0.317 - 02	0.966	0.938	0.957
4.0000 + 05	3.117 - 03	0.316 - 02	0.325 - 02	0.966	0.928	0.954
5.0000 + 05	3.137 - 03	0.136 - 02	0.327 - 02	0.966	0.928	0.957
6.0000 + 05	3.123 - 03	0.315 - 02	0.326 - 02	0.966	0.925	0.957
8.0000 + 05	3.049 - 03	0.306 - 02	0.318 - 02	0.965	0.920	0.956
1.0000 + 06	2.950 - 03	0.297 - 02	0.308 - 02	0.965	0.922	0.956
1.5000 + 06	2.693 - 03	0.270 - 02	0.281 - 02	0.964	0.920	0.958
2.0000 + 06	2.476 - 03	0.248 - 02	0.257 - 02	0.968	0.921	0.954
3.0000 + 06	2.160 - 03	0.219 - 02	0.225 - 02	0.962	0.928	0.954
4.0000 + 06	1.950 - 03	0.199 - 02	0.203 - 02	0.958	0.930	0.948
5.0000 + 06	1.801 - 03	0.186 - 02	0.188 - 02	0.954	0.934	0.944
6.0000 + 06	1.691 - 03	0.178 - 02	0.178 - 02	0.960	0.940	0.949
8.0000 + 06	1.541 - 03	0.165 - 02	0.163 - 02	0.958	0.950	0.944
1.0000 + 07	1.445 - 03	0.159 - 02	0.154 - 02	0.935	0.960	0.929
1.5000 + 07	1.313 - 03					
2.0000 + 07	1.251 - 03					

where:

$$f = (0.876)\ \frac{(\mu_{en}/\rho)_{medium}}{(\mu_{en}/\rho)_{air}}\ (cGy/R)$$

Note: The notation 1.000 ± 4 stands for 1×10^4.

1.13 Human Tissues

1.13.1 Elemental Composition, Atomic Number, and Atomic Mass of Significant Components in Grams of Selected Human Tissue and Organs, Referenced to Water[7,11]

Element	Atomic Number	Atomic Mass	Organ Mass (g) Adipose 15055 g	Blood 5394 g	Brain 1400 g
Calcium	20	40.08	3.4 - 01	3.1 - 01	1.2 - 01
Carbon	6	12.01	9.6 + 03	5.4 + 02	1.7 + 02
Chlorine	17	35.453	1.8 + 01	1.5 + 01	3.2 + 00
Hydrogen	1	1.00797	1.8 + 03	5.5 + 02	1.5 + 02
Iron	26	55.847	3.6 - 01	2.5 + 00	7.4 - 02
Magnesium	12	24.305	3.0 - 01	2.1 - 01	2.1 - 01
Nitrogen	7	14.0067	1.2 + 02	1.6 + 02	1.8 + 01
Oxygen	8	15.9994	3.5 + 03	4.1 + 03	1.0 + 03
Phosphorus	15	30.9738	2.2 + 00	1.9 + 00	4.8 + 00
Potassium	19	39.102	4.8 + 00	8.8 + 00	4.2 + 00
Sodium	11	22.9899	7.6 + 00	1.0 + 01	2.5 + 00
Sulfur	16	32.064	1.1 + 00	5.5 + 00	2.4 + 00
Zinc	30	65.37	2.7 - 02	3.4 - 02	1.7 - 02

Organ Mass (g)

Heart 330 g	Kidney 310 g	Liver 1800 g	Muscle 28,000 g	Pancreas 100 g	Water 1 g
1.2 - 02	2.9 - 02	9.0 - 02	8.7 - 01	9.1 - 03	
5.4 + 01	4.0 + 01	2.6 + 02	3.0 + 03	1.3 + 01	
5.4 - 01	7.4 - 01	3.6 + 00	2.2 + 01	1.6 - 01	
3.4 + 01	3.2 + 01	1.8 + 02	2.8 + 03	9.7 + 00	0.111901
1.5 - 02	2.3 - 02	3.2 - 01	1.1 + 00	3.9 - 03	
5.4 - 02	4.0 - 02	3.1 - 01	5.3 + 00	1.6 - 02	
8.8 + 00	8.5 + 00	5.1 + 01	7.7 + 02	2.1 + 00	
2.3 + 02	2.3 + 02	1.2 + 03	2.1 + 04	6.7 + 01	0.888099
4.8 - 01	5.0 - 01	4.7 + 00	5.0 + 01	2.3 - 01	
7.2 - 01	5.9 - 01	4.5 + 00	8.4 + 01	2.3 - 01	
4.0 + 00	6.2 - 01	1.8 + 00	2.1 + 01	1.4 - 01	
5.4 - 01	0.0 + 00	5.2 + 00	6.7 + 01		
8.4 - 03	1.5 - 02	8.5 - 02	1.5 + 00	2.5 - 03	

Note: The notation 1.00 ± 02, for example, stands for 1.00×10^2.

1.13.2 Mass of the Organs of the Standard Adult Human Body[13]

Tissue or organ	Mass[a] (g)	% of total body
Adipose tissue	15000	21
Subcutaneous	7500	11
Other separable	5000	7.1
Interstitial	1000	1.4
Yellow marrow (included with		
skeleton	1500	2.1
Adrenals (2)	14	0.02
Aorta	100	0.14
Contents (blood)	190 (180 ml)	0.27
Blood-total	5500 g (5200 ml)	7.8
Plasma	3100 g (3000 ml)	4.4
Erythrocytes	2400 g (2200 ml)	3.4
Blood vessels (not including		
aorta and pulmonary)	200 (2900 ml)	0.29
Contents (blood)	3000	4.3
Cartilage (included with skeleton)	1100	1.6
Connective tissue	3400	4.8
Tendons and fascia	1400	2.0
Periarticular tissue	1500	2.1
Other connective tissue	500	0.7
Separable connective tissue	1600	2.3
Central Nervous System	1430	2.04
Brain	1400	2.0
Spinal cord	30	0.04
Contents—cerebrospinal fluid	120 (120 ml)	0.17
Connective tissue	15	0.02
Eyes		
Lenses (2)	0.4	
Gall bladder	10	0.01
Contents (bile)	62 (60 ml)	0.09
GI tract	1200	1.7
Esophagus	40	0.06
Stomach	150	0.21
Intestine	1000	1.4
Small	640	0.91
Upper large	210	0.30
Lower large	160	0.23
Contents of GI tract	1005	1.4
(food plus digestive fluids)		
Hair	20	0.03
Heart	330	0.47
Contents (blood)	500 (470 ml)	0.71
Kidneys	310	0.44
Larynx	28	0.04
Liver	1800	2.6
Lungs	1000	1.4
Parenchyma (includes bronchial		
tree, capillary blood, and		
associated lymph nodes)	570	0.81

1.13.2 Mass of the Organs of the Standard Adult Human Body[13] (continued)

Tissue or Organ	Mass[a] (g)	% of total body
Pulmonary blood	430 (400 ml)	0.61
Lymphocytes	1500	2.1
Lymphatic tissue	700	1.0
Lymph nodes (dissectible)	250	0.36
Miscellaneous (by difference)	2953.1	4.2
Soft tissue (nasopharnyx, etc.)	300	0.43
Fluids (synovial, pleural, etc.)	350	0.50
Muscle (skeletal)	28,000	40.0
Nails	3	
Pancreas	100	0.14
Parathyroids	0.12	
Pineal	0.18	
Pituitary	0.6	
Prostate	16	0.023
Salivary Glands	85	0.12
Skeleton	10,000	14
Bone	5000	7.2
Cortical	4000	5.7
Trabecular	1000	1.4
Red Marrow	1500	2.1
Yellow Marrow	1500	2.1
Cartilage	1100	1.6
Periarticular tissue (skeletal)	900	1.3
Skin	2600	3.7
Epidermis	100	0.14
Dermis	2500	3.6
Hypodermis	7500	11
Spleen	180	0.26
Teeth	46	0.066
Testes	35	0.05
Thymus	20	0.029
Thyroid	20	0.029
Tongue	70	0.10
Tonsils	4	0.006
Trachea	10	0.014
Ureters	16	0.023
Urethra	10	0.014
Urinary bladder	45	0.064
Contents (urine)	102 (100 ml)	0.15
Total body	70,000	100

[a]Values for organs and tissues listed in the right hand column under "Mass" make up the totality of Reference Man (70,000 g).

1.13.3 Chemical Composition of the 70 kg Adult Human Body[13]

Element	Amount (g)	Percent of total body weight
Oxygen	43,000	61.0
Carbon	16,000	23.0
Hydrogen	7000	10.0
Nitrogen	1800	2.6
Calcium	1000	1.4
Phosphorus	780	1.1
Sulfur	140	0.20
Potassium	140	0.20
Sodium	100	0.14
Chlorine	95	0.12
Magnesium	19	0.027
Silicon	18	0.026
Iron	4.2	0.006
Fluorine	2.6	0.0037
Zinc	2.3	0.0033
Rubidium	0.32	0.00046
Strontium	0.32	0.00046
Bromine	0.20	0.00029
Lead	0.12	0.00017
Copper	0.072	0.00010
Aluminum	0.061	0.00009
Cadmium	0.050	0.00007
Boron	<0.048	0.00007
Barium	0.022	0.00003
Tin	<0.017	0.00002
Manganese	0.012	0.00002
Iodine	0.013	0.00002
Nickel	0.010	0.00001
Gold	<0.010	0.00001
Molybdenum	<0.0093	0.00001
Chromium	<0.0018	0.000003
Cesium	0.0015	0.000002
Cobalt	0.0015	0.000002
Uranium	0.00009	0.0000001
Beryllium	0.000036	
Radium	3.1×10^{-11}	

1.14 Tolerance of Selected Organs and Tissues to Ionizing Radiation

(Tissue tolerance figures are constantly being refined as new data become available; figures below are to be used only as guidelines.)

Eye	5-10 Gy, early cataracts, blocked tear ducts from fibrosis. Above 45 Gy to optic nerve/optic chiasm can result in early loss of vision.
Mucosa	20 Gy, erythema, followed by radiation mucositis at higher doses.
Breast	Child, 10-15 Gy, inhibited development, may cause malignancy. Adult, > 60 Gy skin changes and fibrosis.
Heart	Pericarditis above 45 Gy to most of pericardium.
Pelvis	Contains 25% of functional bone marrow in adults; limit area.
Genital Organs	Sterility after 15-20 Gy to ovary or testes. Male, wait 6-8 weeks after TUR to avoid stenosis.
Small Intestine	GI problem at 20-25 Gy. Doses > 45 Gy to large field can result in adhesions
Pancreas	Not dose limiting.
Kidneys	Adult, > 20 Gy to large area can lead to kidney failure, hypertension, uremia, and/ or anemia, requiring transplant. Child, 15 Gy to both, underdevelopment and renal insufficiency.
Lung Parenchyma	20-25 Gy is threshold for pneumonitis, radiation fibrosis prone to infection. Earlier if chemo given concurrently.
Mandible	> 60 Gy, osteonecrosis.
Larynx	> 65 Gy, tissue necrosis.
Thoracic Spine	Upper thoracic spine considered most sensitive, maximum of 45 Gy to limited segmented recommended.
Ribs	> 50 Gy can cause fracture.
Hip joints	> 60 Gy, osteonecrosis of femoral head. Child, > 20 Gy retards bone growth at epiphysis.
Bladder, Urethra, Ureter	> 50 Gy risks hematuria, fibrosis. At 25 Gy, dysuria, but recovery. Above 70 Gy risks fistula. Adjuvant chemotherapy complicates problem.
Rectum, Anus	> 65-70 Gy, tenesmus and ulceration, chronic proctitis requiring colostomy
Spleen	30-40 Gy, loss of immune function.
Adrenals	No record of damage.
Pleura	> 50 Gy may result in painful scarring.
Stomach	15-20 Gy, decrease in hydrochloric acid production. Dose of 40 Gy is well tolerated, but higher risks mucosal ulceration. Large fractions are followed by acute reaction with nausea and vomiting.
Liver	25 Gy threshold in adult for injury; child, 12-25 Gy. If 75% of liver receives 30-35 Gy real risk of liver failure and death. Full blown acute chronic radiation leads to death.

1.14.1 Fetal Dose[14]

Dose in cGy	Risk of Damage
< 5	Low
5 to 10	Uncertain
> 10 to 50	Moderate
> 50	High

1.14.2 Risk by Trimester

	1st	2nd	3rd
> 50 cGy	Highest	Moderate	Low

1.14.3 Normal Tissue Tolerance

TD 5/5, dose producing probability of 5% complication within 5 years; TD 50/5, probability of 50% complication within 5 years; both by fraction of organ volume irradiated[16]

Organ	TD 5/5 Volume 1/3	2/3	3/3
1. Kidney I	5000	3000*	2300
2. Kidney II			
3. Bladder	N/A	8000	6500
4. Bone:			
4A. Femoral Head I and II	—	—	5200
4B. T-M joint mandible	6500	6000	6000
4C. Rib cage	5000	—	—
5. Skin	10 cm²/ - 7000	30 cm²/ - 6000	100 cm²/5000 5500
6. Brain	6000	5000	4500
7. Brain Stem	6000	5300	5000
8. Optic nerve I & II	No partial volume	5000	
9. Chiasma	No partial volume	5000	
10. Spinal cord	5 cm/ 5000	10 cm/ 5000	20 cm/ 4700
11. Cauda equina	No volume effect	No volume effect	6000
12. Brachial plexus	6200	6100	6000
13. Eye lens I and II	No partial volume	1000	
14. Eye retina I and II	No partial volume	4500	
15. Ear mid/external	3000	3000	3000*
16. Ear mid/external	5500	5500	5500*
17. Parotid* I and II	—	3200*	3200*
18. Larynx	7900*	7000*	7000*
19. Larynx	—	4500	4500*
20. Lung I	4500	3000	1750
21. Lung II			
22. Heart	6000	4500	4000
23. Esophagus	6000	5800	5500
24. Stomach	6000	5500	5000
25. Small intestine	5000		4000*
26. Colon	5500		4500
27. Rectum	Volume 100 cm³ No volume effect		6000
28. Liver	5000	3500	3000

*<50% of volume dosen't make a significant change.

1.14.1 Normal Tissue Tolerance (continued)

Organ #	TD 50/5 Volume			Selected endpoint
	1/3	2/3	3/3	
1,2	—	4000*	2800	Clinical nephritis
3	N/A	8500	8000	Symptomatic bladder contracture and volume loss
4A	—	—	6500	Necrosis
4B	7700	7200	7200	Marked limitation of joint function
4C	6500	—	—	Pathologic fracture
5	10 cm^2/ -	30 cm^2/ -	100 cm^2/ 6500	Telangiectasia
5	—	—	7000	Necrosis
5				Ulceration
6	7500	6500	6000	Necrosis Infarction
7	—	—	6500	Necrosis Infarction
8	—	—	6500	Blindness
9	No partial volume	No partial volume	6500	Blindness
10	5 cm/ 7000	10 cm/7000	20 cm/ -	Myelitis necrosis
11	No volume effect	No volume effect	7500	Clinically apparent nerve damage
12	7700	7600	7500	Clinically apparent nerve damage
13	—	—	1800	Cataract requiring intervention
14	—	—	6500	Blindness
15	4000	4000	4000*	Acute serous otitis
16	6500	6500	6500*	Chronic serous otitis
17	— (TD 100/5 is 5000)	4600*	4600*	Xerostomia
18	9000*	8000*	8000*	Cartilage necrosis
19	—	—	8000*	Laryngeal edema
20	6500	4000	2450	Pneumonitis
21	7000	5500	5000	Pericarditis
22	7200	7000	6800	Clinical stricture/ perforation
23	7000	6700	6500	Ulceration, perforation
24	6000		5500	Obstruction perforation/fistula
25	6500		5500	Obstruction perforation/ ulceration/fistula
26	Volume 100 cm^3		8000	Severe proctitis/ necrosis/fistula stenosis
27	No volume effect			
28	5500	4500	4000	Liver failure

*<50% of volume dosen't make a significant change.

1.15 Selected Rules of Thumb

1.15.1 Penetration

- Electrons of at least 70 keV are required to penetrate the epidermis (the protective layer of the skin, 0.07 mm thick[12].

- Alpha particles of at least 7.5 MeV are required to penetrate the epidermis.[12]

- Electrons lose energy at a rate of 2 MeV per cm in water. Thus the range in cm is equal to Energy/2. The 80% depth is approximately equal to the Energy/3.

- Electrons lose energy at a rate of 0.274 MeV per meter in air. Thus the range in meters is equal to energy (MeV) $\times$ 3.65.

X or Gamma Rays in Water

		Depth (cm)			
E	HVL	d_{max}	Range		Exit Dose at 20 cm
			(50%)	(20%)	
250 kVp,	3mm Cu	0.0	7.0	16.0	5.0%
Cobalt-60	11mm Pb	0.5	11.5	24.0	24.0%
4 MV	12 mm Pb	1.0	14.5	29.5	35.5%
6 MV	13 mm Pb	1.5	15.5	>33.0	39.0%
10 MV	15 mm Pb	2.5	18.0	>38.0	46.0%
20 MV	15 mm Pb	3.0	21.0	>40.0	52.0%

1.15.2 Distribution of Orbital Electrons

If n represents the level, or orbit number, the number of electrons which reside in each level is:

$$2n^2$$

1.15.3 The Electromagnetic Spectrum

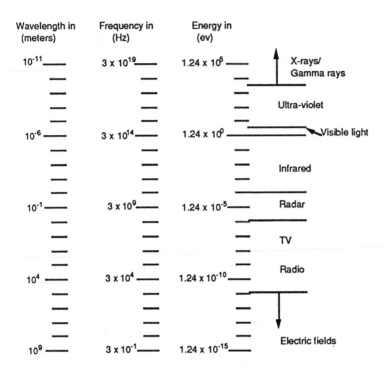

The relationship of photon energy to wavelength is expressed by:

$$E\,(\text{keV}) = \frac{1240}{\lambda\,(\text{picometer})}$$

References to Chapter 1.0

1. *NBS Guidelines for use of the Metric System*, U.S. Department of Commerce, National Bureau of Standards (1977).

2. Cohen, E.R., and Taylor, B.N., The Least-Squares Adjustment of the Fundamental Constants, *J. Phys. Chem. Ref. Data* **2**, 663 (1973).

3. Review of Particle Properties, *Rev. Mod. Phys.* **48**, 2, Part II (1976).

4. Fine, S., and Hendee, W.R., X-Ray Critical Absorption and Emission Energies in keV, *Nucleonics* **13**, 36 (1955).

5. *Physical Aspects Of Irradiation* ICRU Report 10b, International Commission on Radiation Units and Measurements (1964) and NBS Handbook 85, U.S. Government Printing Office, Washington, D.C. (1964).

6. Hagedoorn, H.L, and Wapstra, A.H., Measurements of the Fluorescent Yield of the *K* Shell with a Proportional Counter, *Nucl. Phys.* **15**, (1960).

7. McCullough, E., Photon Attenuation in Computed Tomography, *Med. Phys.* **2**, 307 (1975).

8. Rao, P.S., and Gregg, E.C., Attenuation of Monoenergetic Gamma Rays in Tissues, *Am. J. Roentgenol.***123**, 631 (1975).

9. Hubbell, J.H., *Photon Cross Sections, Attenuation Coefficients and Energy Absorption Coefficients from 10 keV to 100 GeV*, NSDRS-NBS 29, U.S. Government Printing Office, Washington, D.C. (1969).

10. Hubbell, J.H., Photon Mass Attenuation and Mass Energy Absorption Coefficients for H, C, N, O, Ar and Seven Mixtures from 0.1 keV to 20 MeV, *Radiat. Res.* **70**, 58 (1977).

11. Kim, Y.S., Human Tissues: Chemical Composition and Photon Dosimetry Data, *Radiat. Res.* **57**, 38 (1974) and Human Tissues: Chemical Composition and Photon Dosimetry Data. A Correction, *Radiat. Res.* **60**, 361 (1974).

12. *Radiological Health Handbook*, Bureau of Radiological Health, U.S. Public Health Service, Consumer Protection and Environmental Health Service, U.S. Government Printing Service, Washington, D.C. (1970).

13. Snyder,W.S., et al., *Reference Man: Anatomical, Physiological, and Metabolic Characteristics*. Pergamon Press, New York (1975).

14. Pizzarello, D.J., and Witcofski, R.L., *Medical Radiation Biology*, 2nd Ed., Chapter 6, Lea & Febiger, Philadelphia, (1982).

15. Boutillon, Perroche, CCEMRI, Report (I) 85.8, Paris, 1985.

16. Emami, B. et. al: Tolerance of normal tissues to ionizing irradiation, *Int. J. Rad. Oncol. Biol. Physics*, **21** (1) 109, New York, May 1991.

2.0 Teletherapy

2.1 Photons—Kilovoltage

2.1.1 Relationship Between Tube Voltage, Filtration, and Half-Value Layer (HVL)[1]

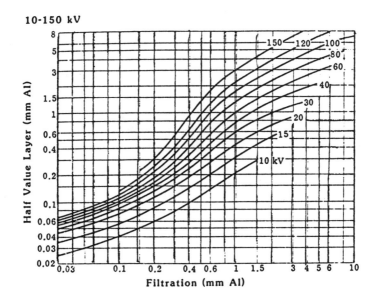

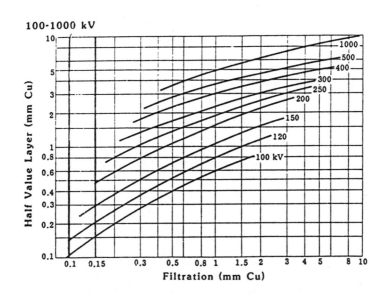

2.1.2 Exposure Rate for Different Voltages and Filtrations[1]

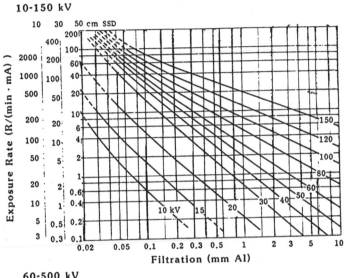

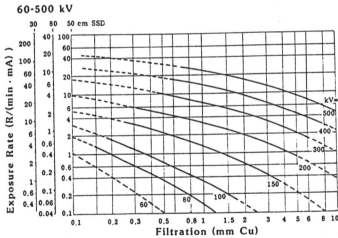

2.1.3 Composition of Thoraeus Filters Used with Orthovoltage X-Rays

Filter	Composition
Thoraeus I	0.2 mm Sn + 0.25 mm Cu + 1 mm Al
Thoraeus II	0.4 mm Sn + 0.25 mm Cu + 1 mm Al
Thoraeus III	0.6 mm Sn + 0.25 mm Cu + 1 mm Al

2.1.4 Temperature-Pressure Correction Factor

Standard laboratories calibrate ionization chambers under atmospheric conditions present in the laboratory and then convert the calibration factor to specific atmospheric conditions—760 mm Hg pressure and 22°C temperature. To correct measurements made under any atmospheric conditions, the following formula can be used:

$$C_{T,P} = \left(\frac{760}{P}\right) \times \left(\frac{273.15 + t}{295.15}\right)$$

where P is the pressure in mm Hg and t is the temperature in °C.

2.1.5 Measurement of Radiation Exposure[2]

Exposure (X) in units of roentgens is measured with a thimble chamber having an exposure calibration factor, N_c, traceable to the National Institute of Science and Technology (NIST; formerly the National Bureau of Standards) for the quality of radiation to be measured:

$$X = M \times N_c \times C_{T,P}$$

where M is the electrometer (chamber) reading and X is the exposure which could be expected in free air at the point of measurement in the absence of the chamber. The roentgen is defined for x- or gamma rays only, and is numerically equal to 2.58×10^{-4} coulombs per kilogram of air at standard temperature and pressure.

2.1.6   Measurement of Radiation Absorbed Dose[3,4]

The original unit of dose was the "rad," an acronym for "radiation absorbed dose." The recommended SI unit is the "gray," which is defined as 1 joule/kilogram, and is numerically equal to 100 rads. Thus one rad is equal to one centigray (cGy).

The absorbed dose in air can be calculated from the measured exposure by use of the factor $W_{air}/e = 33.97$ J/C (average energy absorbed per unit charge of ionization produced in air).

$$\text{Dose (air) (cGy)} = X(\text{C/kg}) \times 33.97 \text{ J/C}$$

Since 1 roentgen $= 2.58 \times 10^{-4}$ C/kg, the dose absorbed in air is equal to:

$$2.58 \times 10^{-4} \times 33.97 \text{ J/C, or } 0.876 \text{ cGy/ R}$$

2.1.7 Absorbed Dose in a Medium

The absorbed dose at a depth in any medium where charged particle equilibrium exists can be calculated from the energy fluence U and the weighted mean mass energy absorption coefficient, μ_{en}/ρ.

$$\text{Dose (D)} = U \times (\mu_{en}/\rho)$$

Let U_{air} represent the energy fluence at a point in air and U_{med} represent the energy fluence at the same point when a medium is interposed in the radiation beam. In the presence of electronic equilibrium for both, the dose in the medium is related to the dose in air as follows:

$$\frac{\text{Dose (med)}}{\text{Dose (air)}} = \frac{\left[\left(\dfrac{\mu_{en}}{\rho}\right)_{med}\right]}{\left(\dfrac{\mu_{en}}{\rho}\right)_{air}} \times \left(\frac{U_{med}}{U_{air}}\right)$$

Since the Dose(air) $= 0.876 \times X(R)$, if we let A equal the ratio of the energy fluences, then:

$$\text{Dose(med)} = 0.876 \times [(\mu_{en}/\rho)_{med}/(\mu_{en}/\rho)_{air}] \times X(R) \times A$$

The quantity in brackets is frequently represented by the symbol f_{med} (also sometimes called the f-factor) so that:

$$\text{Dose (med)} = f_{med} \times X(R) \times A$$

2.1.8 Absorbed Dose to Exposure Ratios for Water and Tissue for Measurements Made at Depth in a Water Phantom[5]

Radiation quality[a]	f(cGy/R) for water	f(cGy/R) for tissue	Radiation quality[a]	f(cGy/R) for water	f(cGy/R) for tissue
0.5 mm Al	0.89	0.91	2 MV	0.95	0.94
1 " "	0.88	0.90	4 MV	0.94	0.93
2 " "	0.87	0.90	6 MV	0.94	0.93
4 " "	0.87	0.90	8 MV	0.93	0.92
6 " "	0.88	0.91	10 MV	0.93	0.91
8 " "	0.89	0.92	12 MV	0.92	0.91
0.5 mm Cu	0.89	0.92	14 MV	0.92	0.91
1.0 " "	0.91	0.93	16 MV	0.91	0.90
1.5 " "	0.93	0.95	18 MV	0.91	0.90
2.0 " "	0.94	0.95	20 MV	0.90	0.89
3.0 " "	0.95	0.95	25 MV	0.90	0.89
4.0 " "	0.96	0.96	30 MV	0.89	0.87
^{137}Cs, ^{60}Co	0.95	0.94	35 MV	0.88	0.86

[a] Half-value layer, nuclide or generating potential in MV corresponding to maximum photon energy are stated to characterize the radiation quality.

2.1.9 Depth Dose Curves in Water or Soft Tissues for Various Quality Beams[6]

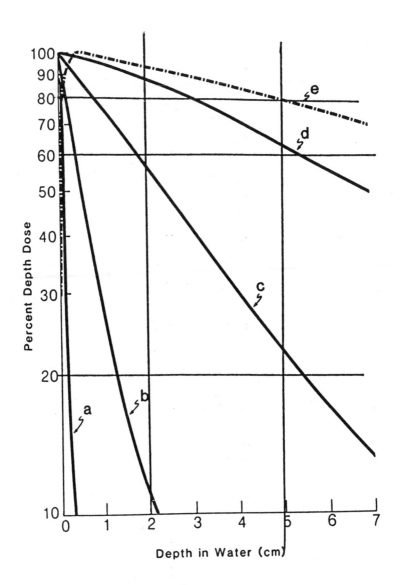

Depth dose curves in water or soft tissues from various quality beams. [Plotted from data in Cohen, M Jones DEA, Green D (eds): *Central Axis Depth Dose Data for Use in Radiotherapy*. Br J Radiol. (Suppl 11) The British Institiute of Radiology, London, 1978.] (a) Grenz rays, HVL = 0.04 mm Al, field diameter ≅ 33 cm, SSD = 10 cm. (b) Contact therapy, HVL = 1.5 mm Al, field diameter = 2.0 cm, SSD = 2 cm. (c) Superficial therapy, HVL = 3.0 mm Al, field diameter = 3.6 cm, SSD = 20 cm. (d) Orthovoltage, HVL = 2.0 mm Cu, field size = 10 × 10 cm, SSD = 50 cm. (e) Cobalt-60 γ rays, field size = 10 × 10 cm, SSD = 80 cm.

2.2 Photons — Megavoltage

2.2.1 AAPM Task Group 21 Calibration Protocol for Photons[7]

The ionization chamber used in this protocol is required to have a ^{60}Co chamber correction factor (N_c, R/C) traceable to the National Institute of Science and Technology (NIST; formerly the National Bureau of Standards). The protocol recommends characterization of the chamber's response by a parameter, N_{gas} (Gy/C) which is a function of a variety of chamber dependent factors. N_{gas} is defined as the dose absorbed in the cavity gas per unit charge, or per unit reading. The ratio of N_{gas} to N_c is a function only of the chamber wall composition and its buildup cap (values of N_{gas}/N_c for a selection of commonly used chambers are published in References 7 and 15. The value of N_{gas} for a chamber can be obtained by multiplying the appropriate value by N_c).

The dose at d_{max} in a medium measured with a chamber without its build-up cap is calculated from an electrometer reading (M) of, say, 200 MU:

$$Dose\ (Gy/MU) = \{M \times N_{gas} \times [aB + (1-a)C] \times p\}/200\ MU$$

where:

1) **a** is the fraction of cavity ionization due to electrons generated in the chamber wall and (1-a) is the fraction generated in the phantom,

2) **B** is the product of two ratios: 1) the average restricted mass collisional stopping power of the electrons in the wall to those in the air, and 2) the average mass energy absorption coefficient of the medium to that of the wall,

3) **C** is the ratio of the average restricted mass collisional stopping power of the electrons in the medium to air, and

4) **p** is the perturbation correction for the change in the electron fluence when the chamber is replaced by the medium.

Values for a, B, C, and p can be obtained from Reference 7.

Also, corrections to the electrometer reading must be made for temperature and pressure, and ion recombination.

2.2.2 Recommended Phantom Depth for Absorbed Dose Calibrations[2]

Type of radiation	Depth (cm)
150 kV - 10 MV x-rays	5
Cobalt-60 Gamma rays	5
11 MV - 25 MV x-rays	7
26 MV - 50 MV x-rays	10

2.2.3 Measurement of Teletherapy Unit Timer Error[8]

Integrate one single exposure of t minutes (R_s),
Integrate multiple exposures (N) of t/N minutes (R_m).

Hence the error = $t [(R_m - R_s)/(NR_s - R_m)]$ minutes.

2.2.4 Approximately Equivalent Squares of Rectangular Fields

The side of an equivalent square field is equal to four times the area of the rectangular field divided by its perimeter. This approximation does not hold for circular or irregular fields; the radius of a circular field with area equal to a rectangular field is:

$$r \cong 4/\sqrt{\pi} \times A/P$$

Equivalent Squares of Rectangular Fields

Axis (cm)	Axis (cm) 2	4	6	8	10	12	14
2	2.0						
4	2.7	4.0					
6	3.1	4.8	6.0				
8	3.4	5.4	6.9	8.0			
10	3.6	5.8	7.5	8.9	10.0		
12	3.7	6.1	8.0	9.6	10.9	12.0	
14	3.8	6.3	8.4	10.1	11.6	12.9	14.0
16	3.9	6.5	8.6	10.5	12.2	13.7	14.9
18	4.0	6.6	8.9	10.8	12.7	14.3	15.7
20	4.0	6.7	9.0	11.1	13.0	14.7	16.3
22	4.0	6.8	9.1	11.3	13.3	15.1	16.8
24	4.1	6.8	9.2	11.5	13.5	15.4	17.2
26	4.1	6.9	9.3	11.6	13.7	15.7	17.5
28	4.1	6.9	9.4	11.7	13.8	15.9	17.8
30	4.1	6.9	9.4	11.7	13.9	16.0	18.0

Axis (cm)	Axis (cm) 16	18	20	22	24	26	28	30
16	16.0							
18	16.9	18.0						
20	17.7	18.9	20.0					
22	18.3	19.7	20.9	22.0				
24	18.8	20.3	21.7	22.9	24.0			
26	19.2	20.9	22.4	23.7	24.9	26.0		
28	19.6	21.3	22.9	24.4	25.7	27.0	28.0	
30	19.9	21.7	23.3	24.9	26.4	27.7	29.0	30.0

2.2.5 Patient Dose Calculation Methods: Fixed Source-Surface Distance (SSD) Technique Versus Isocentric (SAD) Technique [6,10]

2.2.5.1 SSD Technique

Positioning of the patient with the surface to be treated at a fixed distance from the source (commonly at the isocenter of a rotational treatment unit) allows use of previously measured percent depth dose (PDD) tables to calculate either the beam-on time or the monitor units for a given prescribed tumor dose.

PDD tables are constructed from measurements made in a water phantom with the surface maintained at a fixed distance from the source. The probe is positioned along the central axis at successively greater depths and readings are taken for a set interval of time or monitor units. The values at depth are normalized to the point of maximum reading, which is designated the 100% depth, or "d_{max}" depth. It is at this depth the treament unit is calibrated in units of cGy per minute, or cGy per monitor unit.

Since the dose at depth varies with radiation field size, PDD measurements must be made for a selection of clinically useful field sizes. The output at the depth of d_{max} for each field size is normalized to the output for the calibration field size (10×10 cm for x-rays) and a table of field size factors (FSF) is developed.

For example, if a patient were to be treated to a given tumor dose (TD) located at some depth below the surface, the monitor units (MU) set on the machine would be calculated as follows:

$$MU = TD(cGy)/ (PDD \times FSF \times cGy/MU)$$

If an accessory such as a blocking tray or wedge is interposed between the source and the patient, a tray factor or wedge factor would be required in the calculation.

At most institutions, kilovoltage machines are calibrated in air (R/min). It is therefore necessary to convert the output in roentgens to absorbed dose in the phantom by use of a backscatter factor (BSF) which varies with field size, and a cGy/R conversion factor, as illustrated in 2.1.8.

Backscatter factors are measured by comparing the dose measured in air with the dose measured at the same distance from the source but with a sufficient quantity of phantom material to provide full scattering. Backscatter factors vary with field size and the energy of the radiation beam.

Tables of backscatter factors are published in the British Journal of Radiology Supplements.[11]

2.2.5.2 SAD (Isocentric) Technique

Often it is possible to concentrate the radiation dose in the tumor area and spare healthy tissue by delivering the total tumor dose through two or more fields. Accuracy in both positioning the patient and calculating the dose are enhanced by placing the center of the tumor (or target) area at the isocenter, and redirecting the beam by rotating the gantry about the patient. Since the source-axis distance remains constant, this technique is called "isocentric," or the SAD technique.

Because the source-surface distance varies for each field, percent depth dose tables cannot be used. Tables must be developed which represent the dose delivered at a constant distance (at the isocenter) with varying amounts of tissue intervening in the beam, and its relationship to the calibrated output measured at the depth of d_{max} with the surface of the phantom at the isocenter. The values vary with radiation field size, but do not vary with the distance of measurement. These tables are termed Tissue-Output Ratio (TOR) tables. They are developed by positioning the probe at the isocenter, and taking readings at intervals while increasing the depth of the water above the probe. The reading taken at each depth is then divided by the reading taken in the calibration setup.

Using the SAD (isocentric) technique, the monitor unit calculation is made as follows:

$$MU = TD \ (cGy)/ \ [TMR \times cGy/ \ MU]$$

It is important to note that TORs measured in this way (ratioed directly to the calibration setup) do not require what is termed an "inverse square" correction. If, however, the tissue reading is divided by a "calibration reading" taken with the probe at isocenter, then an inverse square correction must be made.

An alternative method is to ratio each measurement made at depth for all field sizes to the maximum reading for that field size (Tissue-Maximum Ratio). In this case, an additional table must be developed of collimator output factors (COF). This factor is measured in air for each field size, and corrects for the fact that output or calibration measurement is made with a 10×10 cm field size.

As with the SSD setup, if accessories are added between the source and the patient, appropriate factors must be used in the monitor unit calculation.

2.3 Photons—General

2.3.1 Atomic Mass and Energy Units[10]

The mass of an atom is expressed in atomic mass units (amu), where one amu is equal to 1.66×10^{-27} kg, one-twelfth the mass of the neutral Carbon-12 atom. From the equation $E = mc^2$, one amu equals 931 MeV.

There are 6.0228×10^{23} atoms are contained in a sample of any element whose weight in grams equals the atomic number of the element. Thus 12 grams of carbon contains 6.0228×10^{23} (Avogadro's number, N_A) atoms, or one gram contains 0.502×10^{23} atoms. The general expression for the number of atoms in one gram of any element is N_A/atomic weight.

2.3.2 Relationship Between the Attenuation Coefficients[10]

Coefficient	Symbol	Relation Between Coefficients	Units of Coefficients	Units in Which Thickness is Measured
linear	μ		m^{-1}	m
mass	(μ/ρ)	μ/ρ	m^2/kg	kg/m^2
electronic	$_e\mu$	$\mu/\rho \times 1/1000\,N_e$	m^2/el	el/m^2
atomic	$_a\mu$	$\mu/\rho \times Z/1000\,N_e$	m^2/at	at/m^2

ρ = density
N_e = number of electons per gram
Z = atomic number of material

2.3.3 Number of Electrons Per Gram for Selected Materials[10]

Material	Density (kg/m^3)	Effective Atomic #	Electrons per Gram
Aluminum	2699	13	2.90×10^{23}
Copper	8960	29	2.75×10^{23}
Lead	11360	82	2.38×10^{23}
Fat	916	6.46	3.34×10^{23}
Water	1000	7.51	3.34×10^{23}
Muscle	1040	7.64	3.31×10^{23}
Bone	1650	12.31	3.19×10^{23}

2.3.4 Relative Importance of Photoelectric (P.E.), Compton (C.), and Pair Production (P.P.) Processes in Water[10]

Radiation Quality (MeV)		Relative Number of Interactions (%)		
Peak Energy	Average Energy	P.E.	C.	P.P.
0.030	0.010	95	5	0
0.080	0.026	60	50	0
0.180	0.060	7	93	0
0.450	0.150	0	100	0
12.0	4.0	0	94	6
30.0	10.0	0	77	23
72.0	24.0	0	50	50
300.0	100	0	16	84

2.3.5 Absorbed Dose to Compact Bone Relative to Soft Tissues for Various Radiation Qualities[10,6]

Radiation Quality		f-Factor		
HVL	Approx. Effective Energy	Muscle cGy/R	Bone cGy/R	Ratio, cGy in bone to cGy in muscle
1 mm Al	20 keV	0.90	4.2	4.7
3 mm Al	30 keV	0.90	4.2	4.7
1 mm Cu	80 keV	0.94	1.9	2.0
2 mm Cu	110 keV	0.95	1.4	1.45
3 mm Cu (250 kVp)	135 keV	0.95	1.1	1.15
10.4 mm Pb (^{60}Co γ ray)	1.25 MeV	0.96	0.92	0.96
11.8 mm Pb (4 MV x-ray)	1.5 MeV	--	--	0.96
14.7 mm Pb (10 MV ")	4 MeV	--	--	0.98
13.7 mm Pb (20 MV ")	8 MeV	--	--	1.02
12.3 mm Pb (40 MV ")	10 MeV	--	--	1.03

2.3.6 Ratio of Linear Attenuation: Bone to Tissue

If the density of bone is assumed to be 1.85 g/cc and that of soft tissue to be 1.0 g/cc, then the attenuation in 1.0 cm of bone will be equivalent to that in 1.65 cm of tissue obtained from the following calculation:

$$\frac{1.85\,(\text{g/cc, bone}) \times 3.00 \times 10^{23}\,(\text{e/cc, bone})}{1.00\,(\text{g/cc, muscle}) \times 3.36 \times 10^{23}\,(\text{e/cc, muscle})} = 1.65\ \text{cm}$$

This increased attenuation has significance in calculating the dose points distal to dense bone.

2.3.7 Thickness of Lead Required to Reduce Useful Beam (Primary Transmission) to 5%[12]

Source type	Energy	Half-value layer (cm)	Required lead[a] (cm)
X-rays	50kV	0.005	0.02
	70kV	0.010	0.04
	100kV	0.025	0.11
	125kV	0.027	0.12
	150kV	0.029	0.13
	200kV	0.042	0.18
	250kV	0.086	0.37
	300kV	0.17	0.73
	2MV	1.15	4.97
	4MV	1.48	6.40
	6MV	1.54	6.66
	8MV	1.62	7.00
	10MV	1.69	7.31
	15MV	1.66	7.18
	20MV	1.63	7.05
	25MV	1.60	6.92
	30MV	1.57	6.79
	40 MV	1.50	6.48
	50 MV	1.43	6.18
Radionuclide	^{60}Co	1.20	5.19
	^{137}Cs	0.65	2.81

[a]Approximate values for broad beams calculated from half-value layers which were obtained or derived from data in ICRP (1982a).

2.3.8 Specifications and Transmissions for Lipowitz's Metal[13,14]

Melting temperature, °F	158
Density, g/cm³	9.4
Specific heat, liquid	0.040
Specific heat, solid	0.040
Latent heat of fusion, BTU/lb	14
Brinell hardness no.	9.2
Tensile strength, lb/in²	5990
% elongation in slow loading	200
Composition, %:	
Bismuth	50
Lead	26.7
Tin	13.3
Cadmium	10

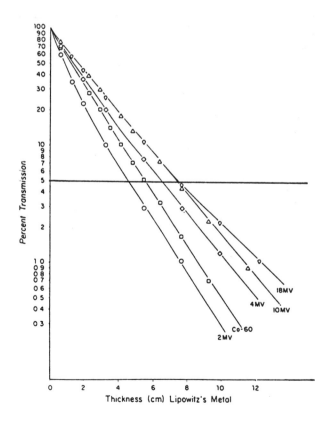

2.3.9 Gap Calculation for Abutting Fields[6]

The gap required to eliminate ovelap and to abut the 50% isodose lines at the midplane (d) of a pair of abutting fields can be calculated as follows:

$$\text{Gap} = s_1 + s_2 = \frac{d}{2} \times \left(\frac{L_1}{SSD_1} + \frac{L_2}{SSD_2} \right)$$

where L_1 and L_2 are the lengths of fields 1 and 2. If one field is significantly larger than the abutted field, a further correction can be made to eliminate the three field overlap which may occur at the depth of the spinal cord. However, this correction usually results in a cold spot at the midplane.

For isocentric SAD setup, if d is the depth of the match point and FS is the field size at the isocenter,

$$s = FS/2 \times d/SAD, \quad \text{and} \quad \text{Gap} = 2s$$

If the abutted fields vary in size, then:

$$\text{Gap} = s_1 + s_2 = \frac{d}{2SAD} \times (FS_1 + FS_2)$$

2.3.10 Comparison of Central Axis Depth Doses in Water for a Wide Variety of Gamma and X-Ray Beams[6]

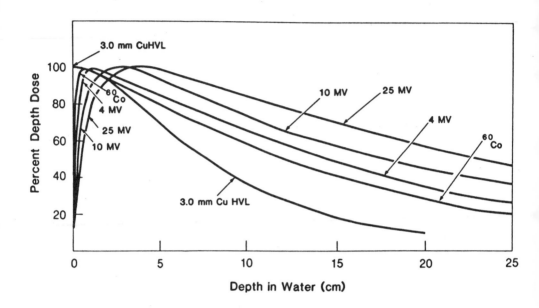

Central axis dose distribution for 10×10 cm field, 100 cm SSD; except for 3.0 mm Cu HVL, SSD = 50 cm.

2.3.11 Wright's Rule of Sevens

- The lateral width of the average human head is 14 cm, with a midplane depth of 7 cm.

- For Cobalt-60 radiation, at 7 cm depth in water, the dose is approximately 70% of the maximum dose.

- For 4 MV x-rays, the dose at 7 cm is approximately 77% of d_{max}.

- A common AP separation for the thorax is 18 cm, with the midplane at nine cm.

- For 10 MV x-rays, the dose at 9 cm is approximately 77% of d_{max}.

2.3.12 Calculation of the Percent Depth Dose Increase with Increase in SSD

The amount of the increase in percent depth dose (PDD) at a fixed depth in water (d) with increase in SSD can be calculated using Mayneord's "f" factor:

$$\text{"f"} = [(SSD_1 + d)/(SSD_1 + d_{max})]^2 \times [(SSD_2 + d_{max})/(SSD_2 + d)]^2$$

then:

$$PDD\ (SSD_2) = \text{"f"} \times PDD\ (SSD_1)$$

2.4 Electrons

2.4.1 AAPM Task Group 21 Calibration Protocol for Electrons[7]

2.4.1.1 Ionization Chamber

Although a parallel plate ionization chamber is the first choice of the protocol (to reduce wall perturbation of the electron field) thimble ionization chambers are commonly used to calibrate electron beams of 4 MeV and above. In either case, a chamber correction factor traceable to the National Institute of Science and Technology (NIST; formerly the National Bureau of Standards) is required.

Farmer type 0.6 cc ionization chambers, with correction applied for perturbation, can be used with acceptable accuracy. Factors for a number of chambers are given in Reference 7.

The position of measurement is displaced 0.75 times the internal radius of the probe, in the direction of the radiation source. Using the N_{gas} method the dose to the medium is:

$$Dose_{med} = M_{med} \times N_{gas} \times (L/\rho)^{med}_{air} \times P_{ion} \times P_{repl}$$

If measurement M is made in water, water replaces medium; however, if measurement is made in plastic, a scattering correction is applied. The chamber is placed in the phantom without the buildup cap, but properly protected in water. Measurement is made at the depth of the maximum dose for each energy. The 15×15 cm electron cone provides an adequate field size for all energies, although the 10×10 cm cone is commonly used at lower energies.

2.4.1.2 Determination of Mean Electron Energy

The mean energy of the beam at the phantom surface is related to the depth at which the dose is 50% of the maximum dose, by the following relationship:

$$\text{Mean energy (MeV)} = 2.33 \times [\text{depth (cm) of } R_{50}]$$

2.4.1.3 Depth of 80% Dose and Range in Water

Because electrons lose about 2 MeV per cm in water, the extrapolated range is approximately one-half the energy. Instructions for determining the extrapolated range are given in Reference 7.

The 80% dose occurs at a depth in cm equal to one-third the value of the energy in MeV.

2.4.2 AAPM Task Group 25 Report on Clinical Electron Beam Dosimetry[13]

The scope of this report has been restricted to two very practical aspects: 1) the description of dosimetry measurement techniques and procedures for acquiring the basic information that is necessary for treatment planning and the acceptance testing of a new electron accelerator and 2) the utilization of dosimetry data for determination of the monitor units required to administer a dose prescription to the patient. The report is too comprehensive to be capsuled; it should be consulted for details. It provides a wealth of bibliographic data for electron beams.

2.4.3 Attenuation Thickness of Lipowitz's Metal

Since electon beams from different manufacturer's linear accelerators vary in mean energy for the same nominal energy, it is recommended each electron beam be measured to determine the thickness of metal required to attenuate the primary beam to 5% at the depth of d_{max} for the open field. The following table is given as a general guide. [15]

		Electron energy (MeV)[a]				
Attenuation	Field size (cm)	6 (6.5)	9 (9.4)	12 (12.8)	16 (16.5)	20 (20.5)
90%	4 × 4	1.8	3.2	4.9	6.8	9.5
	10 × 10	1.9	3.3	4.9	7.0	10.2
	25 × 25	1.9	3.4	5.0	7.7	12.5
93%	4 × 4	2.0	3.7	5.7	9.7	15.7
	10 × 10	2.1	3.8	5.8	10.2	18
	25 × 25	2.1	3.9	6.0	11.3	20.6
95%	4 × 4	2.2	4.3	7.3	16	23.5[b]
	10 × 10	2.3	4.4	8.5	18	25.0[b]
	25 × 25	2.3	4.7	10.0	20	
	4 × 4	2.5	5.5	17.0		
97%	10 × 10	2.8	7.5	19.0		
	25 × 25	2.8	8.0	20.0		

[a]The most probable energy of the incident electron beam as determined by range-energy measurements in a water phantom are given in parentheses directly below the nominal accelerator energies.
[b]Values obtained by linear extrapolation of the bremsstrahlung region.
Note:Table entries are in mm.

References for Chapter 2.0

1. Wachsmann, F. and Drexler, G., *Graphs and Tables for Use in Radiology*. Springer-Verlag, New York (1975).

2. International Commission on Radiological Units and Measurements (ICRU) Report No. 10b: *Physical Aspects of Irradiation*. Washington, D.C., NBS Handbook 85, 1964.

3. ICRU Report No. 33: *Radiation Quantities and Units*. Washington D.C., 1980.

4. ICRU Report No. 31: *Average Energy Required to Produce an Ion Pair*. Washington, D.C., 1979.

5. Saylor, W.S., and Ames, T.C., *Dosage Calculations in Radiation Therapy*, Manual for Univ. of North Carolina, Dept. of Radiology, Chapel Hill, N.C.

6. Kahn, F.M., *The Physics of Radiation Therapy*, Williams and Wilkins, Baltimore/London, 1984.

7. American Association of Physicists in Medicine; RTC Task Group 21: A protocol for the determination of absorbed dose from high energy photon and electron beams. *Med Phys Biol* **10**: 741 (1983).

8. Orton, C.G., et al, The Measurement of Teletherapy Unit Timer Error. *Med Phys Biol* **17**: 202 (1972).

9. Hospital Physicist's Association, Supplement No. 11: *Central axis depth dose data for use in radiotherapy*. British Journal of Radiology, 1978.

10. Johns, H.E. and Cunningham, J.R., *The Physics of Radiology* (3rd Ed.). C.C. Thomas, Springfield, IL (1971).

11. British Journal of Radiology, Suppl. No. 17, *Central Axis Depth Dose Data for Use in Radiotherapy*, London (1983).

12. NCRP Report No. 102: *Medical X-Ray, Electron Beam and Gamma Ray Protection for Energies up to 50 MeV: Equipment Design, Performance and Use*. NCRP, Washington, D.C., 1989.

13. American Association of Physicists in Medicine: RTC Task Group 25: Clinical Electron-Beam Dosimetry: Report of AAPM Radiation Therapy Committee Task Group No. 25., *Med. Physics* **18**(1) Jan/Feb, 1991.

14. Huen, A., et al., Attenuation in Lipowitz's Metal of x-rays Produced at 2, 4, 10, and 18, MV and Gamma Rays from Cobalt-60, *Med. Physics* **6**, 147 (1979).

15. Gasdorf, R., et al., Cylindrical chamber dimensions and the corresponding values of A_{wall} and $N_{gas}/(N \times A_{ion})$. *Medical Physics*, **13**(5), (1986).

3.0 Brachytherapy

3.1 Properties of Radionuclides

3.1.1 Activity

If A is the activity remaining at some time t and A_o is the original activity, then $A = A_0 e^{-\lambda t}$.

$$1 \text{ Ci} = 3.7 \times 10^{10} \text{ Bq}$$

and:

$$1 \text{ bequerel (Bq)} = 1 \text{ dps} = 2.7 \times 10^{-11} \text{ Ci}$$

3.1.2 Mean Life

One half-life $(T_h) = 0.693/\lambda$

The mean life $(T_{avg}) = 1.44 \times T_h$

3.1.3 Physical Properties of Selected Radionuclides[1]

Physical Characteristics of Radionuclides Used in Brachytherapy

Radio-nuclide	Half-life	Photon energy (MeV)	Half-value layer (mm lead)	Exposure rate constant (R-cm²)/(mCi-h)
^{226}Ra	1600 years	0.047-2.45 (0.83 avg)	8.0	8.25*† (R-cm²)/(mg-h)
^{222}Rn	3.83 days	0.047-2.45 (0.83 avg)	8.0	10.15*‡
^{60}Co	5.26 years	1.17, 1.33	11.0	13.07‡
^{137}Cs	30.0 years	0.662	5.5	3.26‡
^{192}Ir	74.2 days	0.136-1.06 (0.38 avg)	2.5	4.69‡
^{198}Au	2.7 days	0.412	2.5	2.38‡
^{125}I	60.2 days	0.028 avg	0.025	1.46‡

* In equlibrium with daughter products.
† Filtered by 0.5 mm Pt.
‡ Unfiltered.

3.2 Transient and Secular Equilibrium[2]

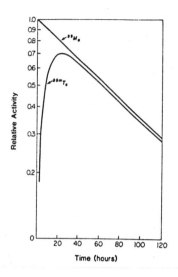

Illustration of transient equilibrium by the decay of ^{99}Mo to ^{99m}Tc. It has been assumed that only 88% of the ^{99}Mo atoms decay to ^{99m}Tc.

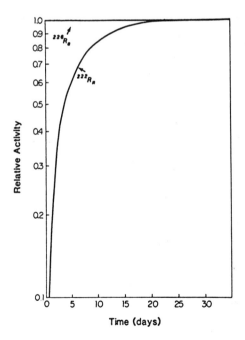

Illustration of secular equilibrium by the decay of ^{226}Ra to ^{222}Rn.

3.3 Linear Source Tables for Radium

Rads per Milligram-Hour in Tissue Delivered at Various Distances by Linear Radium Sources[3]

Filtration = 0.5 mm platinum (Pt). Dose rates are omitted where γ rays traverse more than 7 mm Pt.

Perpendicular Distance from Source (cm)	Distance Along Source Axis (cm from center)				
	0	0.5	1.0	1.5	2.0
	Active Length 1.5 cm				
0.25	50.67	43.75	11.94	3.34	1.48
0.5	20.26	16.95	8.18	3.38	1.70
0.75	10.84	9.29	5.67	2.99	1.67
1.0	6.67	5.89	4.10	2.52	1.55
1.5	3.20	2.96	2.38	1.74	1.24
2.0	1.85	1.76	1.52	1.23	0.96
2.5	1.20	1.15	1.04	0.89	0.74
3.0	0.83	0.81	0.75	0.67	0.58
3.5	0.61	0.60	0.57	0.52	0.46
4.0	0.47	0.46	0.44	0.41	0.37
4.5	0.37	0.36	0.35	0.33	0.30
5.0	0.30	0.29	0.28	0.27	0.25
	Active Length 2.0 cm				
0.25	39.99	37.99	21.38	4.57	1.75
0.5	17.01	15.59	9.97	4.15	1.94
0.75	9.56	8.71	6.14	3.38	1.85
1.0	6.09	5.59	4.23	2.71	1.67
1.5	3.04	2.85	2.37	1.79	1.29
2.0	1.79	1.71	1.51	1.24	0.97
2.5	1.17	1.13	1.03	0.89	0.75
3.0	0.82	0.80	0.75	0.67	0.58
3.5	0.60	0.59	0.56	0.51	0.46
4.0	0.46	0.46	0.44	0.41	0.37
4.5	0.36	0.36	0.35	0.33	0.30
5.0	0.29	0.29	0.28	0.27	0.25
	Active Length 5.0 cm				
0.25	17.29	17.25	—	—	—
0.5	8.21	8.17	8.02	7.66	6.73
0.75	5.15	5.11	4.97	4.66	4.00
1.0	3.62	3.58	3.45	3.20	2.74
1.5	2.10	2.07	1.98	1.82	1.58
2.0	1.37	1.35	1.29	1.19	1.06
2.5	0.96	0.94	0.91	0.84	0.76
3.0	0.70	0.69	0.67	0.63	0.58
3.5	0.54	0.53	0.51	0.49	0.45
4.0	0.42	0.42	0.40	0.38	0.36
4.5	0.34	0.33	0.32	0.31	0.29
5.0	0.27	0.27	0.27	0.26	0.24

Rads per Milligram-Hour in Tissue Delivered at Various Distances by Linear Radium Sources[3] (continued)

Perpendicular Distance from Source (cm)	Distance Along Source Axis (cm from center)					
	2.5	3.0	3.5	4.0	4.5	5.0

Active Length 1.5 cm

	2.5	3.0	3.5	4.0	4.5	5.0
0.25	0.81	0.50	—	—	—	—
0.5	1.00	0.64	0.44	0.31	0.23	0.18
0.75	1.03	0.69	0.48	0.35	0.27	0.21
1.0	1.01	0.69	0.50	0.37	0.28	0.22
1.5	0.89	0.65	0.48	0.37	0.29	0.23
2.0	0.74	0.57	0.45	0.35	0.28	0.23
2.5	0.60	0.49	0.40	0.32	0.26	0.22
3.0	0.49	0.41	0.34	0.29	0.24	0.21
3.5	0.40	0.35	0.30	0.26	0.22	0.19
4.0	0.33	0.29	0.26	0.23	0.20	0.17
4.5	0.28	0.25	0.22	0.20	0.18	0.16
5.0	0.23	0.21	0.19	0.17	0.16	0.14

Active Length 2.0 cm

	2.5	3.0	3.5	4.0	4.5	5.0
0.25	0.90	0.54	—	—	—	—
0.5	1.09	0.68	0.46	0.33	0.24	0.18
0.75	1.11	0.72	0.50	0.37	0.27	0.21
1.0	1.07	0.72	0.51	0.38	0.29	0.23
1.5	0.92	0.67	0.50	0.38	0.30	0.24
2.0	0.75	0.58	0.45	0.36	0.29	0.23
2.5	0.61	0.49	0.40	0.33	0.27	0.22
3.0	0.49	0.42	0.35	0.29	0.25	0.21
3.5	0.40	0.35	0.30	0.26	0.22	0.19
4.0	0.33	0.29	0.26	0.23	0.20	0.17
4.5	0.28	0.25	0.22	0.20	0.18	0.16
5.0	0.23	0.21	0.19	0.17	0.16	0.14

Active Length 5.0 cm

	2.5	3.0	3.5	4.0	4.5	5.0
0.25	—	—	—	—	—	—
0.5	4.31	1.88	0.93	0.55	—	—
0.75	2.80	1.59	0.92	0.58	0.40	0.29
1.0	2.04	1.33	0.86	0.57	0.40	0.30
1.5	1.27	0.96	0.70	0.52	0.39	0.30
2.0	0.89	0.72	0.57	0.45	0.35	0.28
2.5	0.66	0.56	0.47	0.38	0.31	0.26
3.0	0.51	0.45	0.38	0.33	0.27	0.23
3.5	0.41	0.36	0.32	0.28	0.24	0.21
4.0	0.33	0.30	0.27	0.24	0.21	0.18
4.5	0.27	0.25	0.23	0.21	0.18	0.16
5.0	0.23	0.21	0.20	0.18	0.16	0.15

3.4 Dose/Exposure Curves in Water[4]

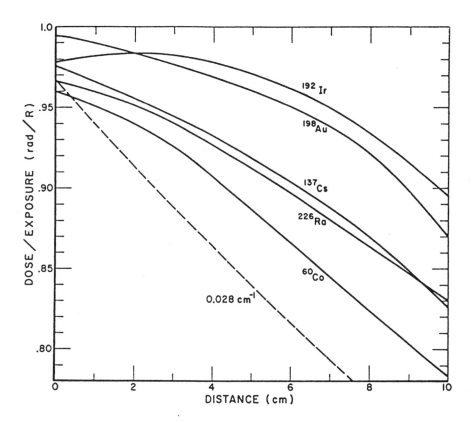

Dose per unit exposure vs. distance for a point source of gamma radiation in water. The ordinates give the ratio of the absorbed dose to water at a given point, to the exposure in air at the same point in the absence of water. The broken curve is calculated for exponential absorption with buildup, using the narrow-beam attenuation coefficient 0.028 cm^{-1}.

3.5 Miscellaneous

3.5.1 Isotope Half-Life in an Organ

$$\frac{1}{T_{effective}} = \frac{1}{T_{physical}} + \frac{1}{T_{biological}}$$

3.5.2 Source Activity

Source activity at the end of 7 half-lives is less than 1%. Ten half-lives reduce source activity by about 1/1000.

References for Chapter 3.0

1. Khan, F. *The Physics of Radiation Therapy*, Williams and Wilkins, Baltimore, M.D., 1984, p. 355.

2. Khan, F. *The Physics of Radiation Therapy*, Williams and Wilkins, Baltimore, M.D., 1984, pp. 20-21.

3. Shalek, R.J. Stovall, M., "Dosimetry in Implant Theray," in *Radiation Dosimetry*, Vol. 3, F.H. Attix, et al., eds. Academic Press, 1969, pp. 761-769.

4. Loevinger, R., Absorbed Dose from Interstitial and Intracavitary Sources, p. 199, in *Proceedings of Afterloading in Radiotherapy*, Simon, N., (Ed.), U.S. HEW 72-8024, Bureau of Radiological Health (1971).

4.0 Radiation Protection

4.1 Radiation Exposure

4.1.1 Dose Equivalents

The dose equivalent (H) is defined as $H = D \times Q \times N$, where D is the absorbed dose, Q is the quality factor for the radiation, and N is the product of all other modifying factors (usually considered as 1.0).

The SI unit for both dose and dose equivalent is J/kg; the special name for H is the sievert (Sv). One Sv is equal to 1 J/kg for x, γ or β radiations.

4.1.2 Quality Factors[1]

Type of radiation	Approximate value of Q
X-rays, gamma rays, beta particles & electrons	1
Thermal neutrons	5
Other neutrons, low energy protons, alpha particles	10

The NRC is currently recommending that a value of 20 be adopted for the particles in the third line, based on actions by the ICRU in 1987.

4.1.3 Natural Background Radiation in the United States[2]

Radiation source	mSv/yr
Cosmic rays	0.28
Terrestrial	0.26
Radionuclides in the body	0.27
Total	0.81

Effective dose equivalent (including lung dose from Radon (Rn) + daughter) = 3.0 mSv (300 mrem).

4.1.4 Critical Organs[3]

For whole-body irradiation, the critical organs are:

    a) gonads, for genetic effects,
    b) bone marrow, for induction of leukemia,
    c) lens of the eye for cataracts; and
    d) skin, for skin cancer

For internally deposited radionuclides, the critical organs are:

    a) thyroid
    b) gastrointesinal tract
    c) lung
    d) bone, and
    e) kidney

4.1.5 NCRP Recommendations for MPDE[1]

Summary of Recommendations[a,b]

A. Occupational exposures (annual)[c]		
1. Effective dose equivalent limit (stochastic effects)	50 mSv	(5 rem)
2. Dose equivalent limits for tissues and organs (nonstochastic effects)		
a. Lens of eye	150 mSv	(15 rem)
b. All others (e.g., red bone marrow, breast, lung, gonads, skin and extremities)	500 mSv	(50 rem)
3. Guidance: cumulative exposure	10 mSv × age	(1 rem × age in yrs)
B. Planned special occupational exposure, effective dose equivalent limit[c]	see Section 15	
C. Guidance for emergency occupational exposure[c]	see Section 16	
D. Public exposures (annual)		
1. Effective dose equivalent limit, continuous or frequent exposure[c]	1 mSv	(0.1 rem)
2. Effective dose equivalent limit, continuous or infrequent exposure[c]	5 mSv	(0.5 rem)
3. Remedial action recommended when:		
a. Effective dose equivalent[d]	>5 mSv	(>0.5 rem)
b. Exposure to radon and its decay products	>0.007 Jhm^{-3}	(>2 WLM)
4. Dose equivalent limits for lens of eye, skin and extremities	50 mSv	(5 rem)
E. Education and training exposures (annual)[c]		
1. Effective dose equivalent limit	1 mSv	(0.1 rem)
2. Dose equivalent limit for lens of eye, skin and extremities	50 mSv	(5 rem)
F. Embryo-fetus exposures[c]		
1. Total dose equivalent limit	5 mSv	(0.5 rem)
2. Dose equivalent limit in a month	0.5 mSv	(0.05 rem)
G. Negligible Individual Risk Level (annual)[c]		
Effective dose equivalent per source or practice	0.01 mSv	(0.001 rem)

[a] Excluding medical exposures.
[b] See 4.1.2 for recommendations on Q.
[c] Sum of external and internal exposures.
[d] Including background but excluding internal exposures.

4.2 Shielding

4.2.1 Photon Transmission Factors Through Lead and Concrete for Selected Beams[4]

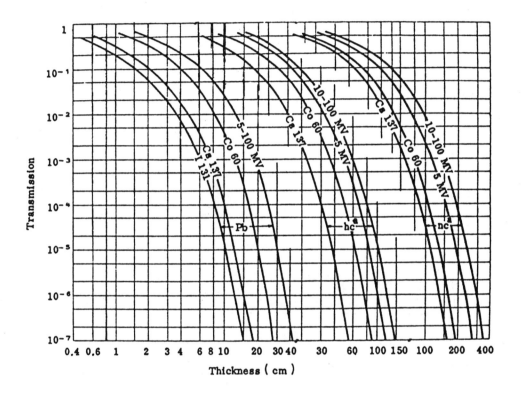

[a]hc - heavy concrete (ρ= 3.2 g/cm^3); nc - normal concrete (ρ= 2.2 g/cm^3)

4.2.2 Average Half-Value and Tenth-Value Layers of Shielding Materials (Broad Beams)[4]

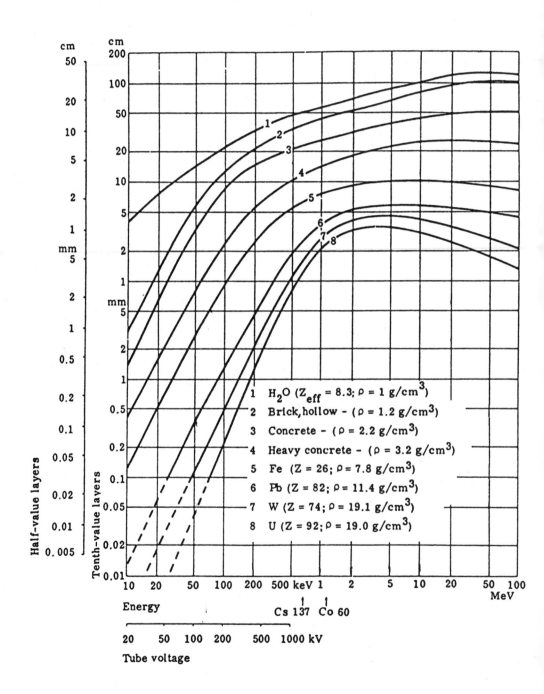

1   H_2O (Z_{eff} = 8.3; ρ = 1 g/cm^3)
2   Brick, hollow – (ρ = 1.2 g/cm^3)
3   Concrete – (ρ = 2.2 g/cm^3)
4   Heavy concrete – (ρ = 3.2 g/cm^3)
5   Fe (Z = 26; ρ = 7.8 g/cm^3)
6   Pb (Z = 82; ρ = 11.4 g/cm^3)
7   W (Z = 74; ρ = 19.1 g/cm^3)
8   U (Z = 92; ρ = 19.0 g/cm^3)

4.2.3 Summary of Measured Fast-Neutron Fluences from Electron Accelerators[5]

Accelerator	Radiation	Energy (MeV)	Field (cm)	SSD(cm)	Target
B.B.C. Betatron	x	32	10 × 10	80	--
B.B.C. Betatron	x	33	25 × 25	100	--
	e⁻	35	25 × 25	110	
M.E.L. Linac	x	16	25 × 25	100	--
B.B.C. Betatron	x	32	10 × 10	100	--
Siemens Betatron	x	19	7.6 × 11.4	50	--
Sagittaire Linac	x	25	10 × 10	100	--
Varian Clinac-18	x	10	10 × 10	100	6.3 mm Cu
Allis Chalmers Betatron	x	25	10 × 10	100	1.6 mm Pt
B.B.C. Betatron	x	45	10 × 10	110	2.0 mm Pt
Varian Clinac-18	x	10	25 × 25	100	Cu
Shimadzu Betatron	x	18	20 × 20	100	2 mm Pt
	x	23	20 × 20	100	2 mm Pt
	x	23	10 × 10	100	2 mm Pt
	e⁻	25	14 × 14	105	

4.2.3 Summary of Measured Fast-Neutron Fluences from Electron Accelerators[5] (continued)

Accelerator	Beam filter	Inside field per rad of x-rays or electrons	Neutron fluence (distance outside field edges) $(10^4 \text{ cm}^{-2} \text{ rad}^{-1})$ (uncertainty)		Outside field
B.B.C. Betatron	—	0.51	0.18		(0-7 cm)
B.B.C. Betatron	—	18 (30%-40%)	5.0	(±35%)	(27.5 cm)
	—	0.66 (30%-40%)	0.29	(±35%)	(27.5 cm)
M.E.L. Linac	—	15 (30%-40%)	7.1	(±35%)	(27.5 cm)
B.B.C. Betatron	—	130 (-)	85	(-)	(5 cm)
Siemens Betatron	—	73 (±15%)	17		(5 cm)
Sagittaire Linac	—	180 (±10%)	28		(5 cm)
Varian Clinac-18	W	1.06 (±20%)	1.52	(±20%)	(5 cm)
Allis Chalmers Betatron	Al	13.6 (±20%)	10.1	(±20%)	(5 cm)
B.B.C Betatron	Pb	14.4 (±20%)	10.0	(±20%)	(5 cm)
Varian Clinac-18	W		0.4 (factor of ~2)		(100 cm)
Shimadzu Betatron	413 g Pb	4.8 (±50%)			
	413 g Pb	6.2 (±50%)	2.9	(±50%)	(5 cm)
			1.0	(±50%)	(20 cm)
	413 g Pb	6.0 (±50%)			
	0.3 mm Ta	0.05 (factor of ~2)			

References for Chapter 4.0

1. NCRP Report 91: *Recommendations on Limits for Exposure to Ionizing Radiation*, Washington, D.C., NCRP (1987).

2. NCRP Report 45: *Natural Background Radiation in the Unites States*, Washington, D.C., NCRP (1975).

3. NCRP Report 39: *Basic Radiation Protection Criteria*, Washington, D.C., NCRP (1971).

4. Wacksman, F. et al., *Graphs and Tables for Use in Radiology*, Springer-Verlag, New York (1975).

5. Fox, J.G., et al., Fast Neutrons from a 25 MV Betatron, *Med Phy* **4**: 387 (1979).

5.0 In Vivo Dosimetry

5.1 Thermoluminescent Dosimetry

5.1.1 Characteristics of Various Phosphors[1]

Characteristic	LiF	$Li_2B_4O_7$:Mn	CaF_2:Mn	CaF_2:nat	$CaSO_4$:Mn
Density (g/cc)	2.64	2.3	3.18	3.18	2.61
Effective Atomic #	8.2	7.4	16.3	16.3	15.3
TL emission spectra (A) Range	3500-6000	5300-6300	4400-6000	3500-5000	4500-6000
Maximum	4000	6050	5000	3800	5000
Temperature of main TL glow peak	195°C	200°C	260°C	260°C	110°C
Efficiency at Cobalt-60 (relative to LiF)	1.0	0.3	3	23	70
Energy response without added filter (30 keV/cobalt-60)	1.25	0.9	13	13	10
Useful range	mR-10^5 R	mR-10^6 R	mR-3×10^5 R	mR-10^4 R	R-10^4 R
Fading	Small, <5%/12 wk	10% in first month	10% in first month	No detectable fading	50-60% in the first 24 hrs.
Light sensitivity	Essentially none	Essentially none	Essentially none	Yes	Yes
Physical form	Powder, extruded, Teflon-embedded, silicon-embedded, glass capillaries	Powder, Teflon-embedded	Powder, Teflon-embedded, hot-pressed chips, glass capillaries	Special dosimeters	Powder, Teflon-embedded

References for Chapter 5.0

1. Cameron, J.R., et al: *Thermoluminescent Dosimetry*, Madison, WI, University of Wisconsin Press (1968).

Acknowledgment

I am deeply grateful to John Horton, who took time from a very busy schedule to review my manuscript and then made very helpful suggestions.